DARE
TO BE AWESOME

How to Design the Life of Your
Dreams One Habit at a Time

DEE MATLOK

First published by Ultimate World Publishing 2021
Copyright © 2021 Dee Matlok

ISBN

Paperback: 978-1-922597-77-9
Ebook: 978-1-922597-78-6

Cover design: Ultimate World Publishing
Layout and typesetting: Ultimate World Publishing
Editor: James Salmon
Cover photo copyright license: Kair-Shutterstock.com

Ultimate World Publishing
Diamond Creek,
Victoria Australia 3089
www.writeabook.com.au

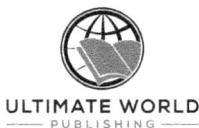

Disclaimer

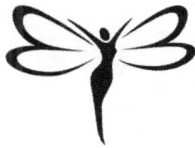

The statements and opinions expressed in this book are for educational purposes only and are not intended as a substitute for professional advice that may be specific to your needs and circumstances. Mentions of any individuals, companies, products, or services are for illustration purposes only and should not be considered as a recommendation.

Contents

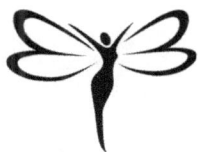

Introduction

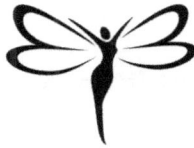

Background

The idea for this book was formed in 2020, the year that the COVID-19 pandemic dramatically disrupted our lives. There were lockdowns, restrictions on gatherings, mandatory wearing of face masks in public places, and sadly, many deaths. If 2020 taught me anything, it was that life can change quickly and unexpectedly and that plans such as that overseas holiday or celebrating birthdays with my parents were no longer a given. What if I never get to see my parents again? What if I have to wait another two years or more before I can see my friends and family who live thousands of kilometres away? What if I never get a chance to visit all those countries I have always wanted to visit but have kept putting it off?

I have always been a very organised and driven person. If I put my mind to achieving something I generally achieve it. I don't think I have any particular talents or skills, but when I want to achieve something, I do apply myself to the task and goal. Importantly, I have also set myself up with positive habits that help support me on my life's journey and that increase the likelihood that I will meet my goals. Yet over the years, I have met many people who for whatever reason felt stuck in their lives and weren't able to achieve their goals. Goals such as weight loss, eating healthier, saving more money or getting better quality sleep. People struggling to stick with habits and therefore not reaching goals they have set for themselves to have a better life.

Why you should read this book

"The trajectory of your life bends in the direction of your habits."

James Clear

There may be any number of reasons why you have picked up this book.

You may be successful in your work, in raising your family, or in other areas of your life such as contributing to the community, but somehow, you have forgotten to look after yourself and be the best you can be.

You are feeling stuck in your life – poor diet, unfit or unhealthy, not saving as much money as you would like – and you want to make a change but don't know how to.

You've tried to make changes in the past but have not succeeded.

Many of us care for people in our lives such as partners, children, and parents. We only want what is best for them. We nurture them and encourage them to be their best. We feed our pets premium pet food. We also take care of physical assets in our life such as our house and motor vehicle. But we do not seem to extend that same care and attention to ourselves. It's the classic story of the mechanic who drives a beaten up and unreliable car or the doctor who is in ill health. We care for others but don't hold ourselves to that same standard. And we should. That is not being selfish.

One of the books that I read when I was in the corporate world was a book called Strategy and the Fat Smoker by David Meister. While the focus of the book is on corporate strategy, its main idea applies to our personal lives as well; that we often know what we should be doing to be successful but it is not always easy to do. In our personal lives, we often know what we need to do to improve – to eat healthier, to exercise more, to get more sleep – but we don't always follow through with those goals.

This book presents ideas on how you can implement positive change in key areas of your personal life through the formation and maintenance of positive habits and how to help make those habits stick.

What does the dragonfly image mean?

The symbol on the cover represents a powerful and evolving dragonfly and is the symbol of my business. Dragonflies are amazing creatures. They moult many times throughout their life, shedding the old and taking on the new. Each phase that it goes through symbolises growth and change. As the dragonfly evolves, it becomes stronger and more beautiful. In essence, the dragonfly represents strength, beauty and positive change and symbolises life lived to the fullest.

Are you ready to live your life to the fullest, create positive habits that stick, and design the life of your dreams?

How to use this book

This book is designed to give you practical ideas on how to implement changes in your daily life to create a better version of you.

Most people don't create their life in a way to make good habits easier to practise. Throughout this book I will be sharing ideas on some actionable things you can do to design your awesome life.

Chapter 1 explains what habits are and introduces the DARE Model of habit formation.

Chapter 2 presents you with exercises and tools to evaluate your current lifestyle and determine where you want to be.

Chapter 3 identifies ways to delete anything from your life that is unnecessary.

My research and my conversations with people have indicated that there are main areas where people are seeking to improve their lives and lifestyle. To eat healthier. To exercise more. To save more money. To get better sleep. So, Chapters 4 to 11 focus on those lifestyle areas where people desire a level of improvement. For example, the chapter called "Nourish" is to help people to eat healthier. The chapter called "Rest" is to help people get a better night's sleep. I call these the lifestyle chapters and each one is self-contained and focuses on a particular area of our lives that we often strive to improve but don't always achieve. While each chapter can be read on its own, you are encouraged to read the book right through from the beginning to the end as advice and tips in one chapter may be applicable to other areas of your life. Each lifestyle chapter takes you through some ideas on how you can improve that particular area of your life and ends with a sample of a completed DARE template to prompt you with ideas on how to apply the DARE Model in your own life. The Appendix has a blank DARE template that you can also download from www.deematlok. com. The website also has other ideas and resources to help you form good habits, and there are bonus offers that are available on the website.

CHAPTER 1

DARE

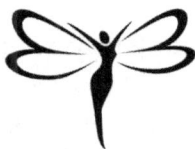

"We first make our habits, then our habits make us."
John Dryden

What is a habit?

So, what exactly is a habit?

The Macquarie Dictionary defines a habit as a particular practice or custom, a tendency to act in a certain way, acquired by frequent repetition of an act. Think about some of the things that you do every day without giving it any thought. It might be making your morning coffee, having a shower, brushing your teeth, or driving your car out of your garage. How many times have you done those things without giving any thought to that activity? That is a habit. A habit is something that is so ingrained that it doesn't require any thought.

Habits are behaviours that are wired deep in our brains so that we perform them automatically. They are things you really don't have to think about. A significant part of our day is made up of habitual actions that we do on autopilot. Applying makeup, taking your children to school, even the smallest actions such as automatically putting on your seatbelt when you get into a car and then driving to work. Think back to the first few times that you drove to somewhere you regularly go, such as your place of work. You probably spent time actively thinking about the route and paying attention to your surroundings. But the repetition of that action over time started to embed this as a habit. Fast forward to today and there may be times when you have driven to work and you don't recall a large part of that journey, as you were on autopilot. This allows you to follow the same route to work every day without thinking about it, freeing up your mind to consider other things, such as what to make for dinner.

The idea behind developing good habits is that firstly, you can automate positive behaviours that support your goals (such as eating more vegetables to be healthier) and secondly, it reduces the mental toll that making decisions can bring. If we didn't form habits, the mental burden of having to actively think about all these daily tasks would be exhausting. The value of a habit is that you don't have to think about it and it can then free up your brain to do other things.

Aren't habits just about repetition?

> *"We are what we repeatedly do. Excellence, then is not an act but a habit."*
>
> Aristotle

This is such a powerful quote. You can imagine, think, believe, plan and prepare as much as you like, but all of that mental thought is only part of the story of success. You also need to 'do'. We are what we repeatedly do. Did you eat a healthy lunch that you prepared in the morning, or did you hit the snooze button and end up eating a calorie-laden takeaway for lunch? Did you slouch on the couch in the evening, drinking wine, or did you exercise for twenty minutes?

There's a popular belief that you need to practise your habit for a certain number of days before it is embedded, but the current thinking is that it is less to do with the number of days and more to do with other factors, such as your mindset and your environment. It will also depend on the simplicity or complexity of the habit you are trying to create. A simple habit may only take a few repetitions to become automated while a more complex habit could take longer to ingrain. Think of any of the skills-based sports such as gymnastics or golf. It takes many years and countless repetitions to learn, perfect and automate movements such as a golf swing or an aerial cartwheel.

Getting habits to stick is also a product of the environment that you create, not just the repetition of the action. It is also influenced by your mindset. We say things to ourselves like "I'm a terrible cook", or "I'm not a morning person" and over time that becomes part of your identity and you accept them without ever challenging them. When you cook an ordinary meal or struggle to wake in the morning, this then reinforces that belief. If you want to make a change in your life, a key element is that you need to shift your mindset as well.

What about willpower?

Willpower is the ability to resist temptation and delay gratification in order to meet long-term goals. Exercising willpower requires vigilance though, which can be exhausting and accordingly willpower will only last for so long. I'm sure you've experienced this in some form, such as trying to stick to a healthy diet and then being tempted to order a large calorie-rich dessert at the end of an otherwise satisfying meal. You may have wanted to avoid dessert as part of your goal of sticking to a healthy diet but perhaps your willpower failed you. And what about good intentions? Many people decide on 31 December that they will implement a number of New Year's resolutions in the following year. They are full of good intentions and hopes and dreams. But studies show that by February, 80% of people have already started to falter or have given up on those resolutions. However, developing good habits means you are less reliant on willpower and intentions.

You also can't rely on willpower, particularly later in the day. We make so many decisions every day that our ability to make smart choices tends to deteriorate as the day wears on. This is one of the reasons why we can eat well all day but then fall off the wagon in the evening, reaching for that chocolate or large glass of wine. Motivation, discipline and willpower do not always work as they are energy-sapping.

While motivation, willpower and good intentions are great, they don't always transfer into action. Sometimes action has to precede the motivation. Taking a small step in the direction that you want to go can build momentum. For example, putting on your running shoes to go for a run can be enough to motivate you to get out the door and go for that run. If you start with an action, then the motivated feeling will usually follow.

Many people are of the belief that they are unable to achieve their goals due to lack of motivation. In reality, it is more likely to be due to a number of other factors. Not being clear on your goal is one example, and goals need to be SMART. SMART stands for Specific, Measurable, Achievable, Relevant and Time-based. SMART goals should also be stated positively and in the present tense, as if you have already achieved the goal. For example, "It is 3 April 2021 and I am getting 7 ½ hours of quality sleep a night". SMART Goals are discussed in more detail in Chapter 2.

What tactics have you used to create a habit?

At some time in your adult life, you have probably had to take a course of prescription medication, such as antibiotics. Such medications are usually required to be taken regularly, for example twice daily with meals. How did you remember to take your medication? Did you set a reminder? Did you place the medication in a visible location to remind you to take it? Did you put it next to your coffee pods or tea bags to remind you to take it with your breakfast? Think about the tactics you have employed and how you can apply that process to build other habits into your life.

The key elements to forming good habits

In their popular books, authors Charles Duhigg[1] and James Clear[2] unpack the ways how and the reasons why habits are formed.

Duhigg states that there are three key elements to forming a habit, which he calls the habit loop. The habit loop is a basic framework that helps explain, in simple terms, how a habit is formed. Duhigg describes those elements of the habit loop as:

(i) Cue – this is a trigger that causes a habit to start automatically, such as a location, a time of day, an emotion or a person. For example, a trigger may be where every day at 10.00 am you crave a cup of coffee.

(ii) Routine – this is the most obvious part of a habit as this is the repeated behaviour that is automatic. So for example, when the cue of craving a cup of coffee at 10.00 am happens, you join a colleague for a coffee and a chocolate biscuit.

(iii) Reward – this is what the behaviour or routine does for you, so for example, when you have the coffee and biscuit with your colleague, you get a caffeine hit, a sugar hit, as well as the benefits of a social connection.

Below is an image that shows the habit loop:

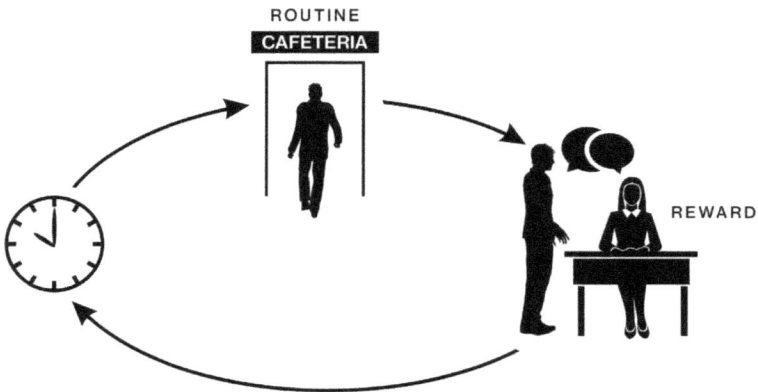

Image 1a – habit loop

More recently, Clear explains that there are four simple rules for building better habits. They are:

(a) make it obvious
(b) make it attractive
(c) make it easy, and
(d) make it satisfying.

And to eliminate bad habits, do the opposite, in other words:

(a) make it invisible
(b) make it difficult
(c) make it unattractive, and
(d) make it unsatisfactory.

My views on habits are largely in line with the works of Duhigg and Clear, however I am not convinced that a habit needs to be easy, at least not in the beginning. Any behavioural change is an adjustment to the way you live your life, and humans are creatures of comfort. Change can be hard, especially if you are trying to undo years of bad habits, or if you don't have support around you. It isn't always easy to make a change, so don't be too hard on yourself if you struggle at times. Every new beginning can be challenging and hard. But over time, it can and does get easier.

> *"Every action is a vote for the type of person you wish to become."*
>
> James Clear

Clear also states that there are two main factors that contribute to habit change and they are identity change and environment change.

Identity change is deciding on the type of person you want to be and focussing not on what you want to achieve but on who you want to become.

13

Clear also focusses on the changes you need to make to your environment in order to make any new habit easier to do.

"The more disciplined your environment is, the less disciplined you need to be. Don't swim upstream."
James Clear

DARE Model

"Life is short, they say. But maybe it's just long enough if you live it right."
Unknown

The works of Duhigg, Clear and countless others have made significant contributions to the fields of psychology and behavioural science and have influenced how we, as individuals, can improve our lives by gaining a better understanding of how habits are formed and ingrained. However, through my research and conversations with people, I realised that many of them simply needed some practical guidance on how to create and maintain positive habits.

The title of this book is meant to not only challenge you to be your best – to dare to be awesome – but it is also a reference to an acronym of the four simple and practical elements that I believe are essential to ensure that the positive habits you want to establish will stick and endure.

My model for helping habits stick is called DARE, which is an acronym for Desire, Accountability, Reward, and Environment.

"Before you can change your world, you have to believe that you can change it."

Amy Morin

Desire

Firstly, you must want to make a shift and a change in your life. Intention is one thing, but it is not enough. You need a deep-seated desire to drive you forward into making a change. For example, if you want to start exercising, your reason is likely to be because you want to get fitter and healthier, not because you want to exercise more.

So, what is your 'why'?

Achieving any goal requires you to ask this fundamental question. Why do you want to achieve this goal? Having a meaningful reason for achieving your goal is a key factor in your success. For example, you may wish to lose weight. What is your reason? Is it aesthetics? Or is it to have more energy to play with your children or your grandchildren? Or is it to tackle a health risk such as type 2 diabetes? Whatever your goal, the more meaningful it is, the greater your desire for achieving it will be, and the more likely you are to succeed in achieving your goal.

"...true behaviour change is identity change. Every action you take towards your goal is a vote for the person you wish to become. You're no longer that someone who tries to go for a run three times a week, you're a runner. We can all begin by asking ourselves, 'Who do I want to become?'"[3]

You have to have the desire to change. Not just change your behaviour, but also change your identity.

You need to also evaluate how you talk to yourself and the language you use. Some of us hold onto beliefs about ourselves that are limiting, such as "I am a terrible cook", or "I am hopeless at maths". But have you internalised those statements and do you actually believe them? If you do, then you risk being stuck in an ongoing rut. However, these limiting beliefs don't need to be fixed for life. We are all capable of improving our lives significantly if we can identify and change such limiting beliefs. The next time a limiting belief presents itself, challenge its validity. Is there any truth to that belief or is it another person's opinion?

Another key element to success is cultivating a positive mindset, imagining what is possible, rather than thinking about what could go wrong. Ask yourself questions such as "What is possible if I do this?" Focus on what you do want, rather than what you don't want.

We are also capable of making excuses. We say things like:

- I'm too busy
- I'm too tired
- I don't have enough money

While we all make excuses as to why we can't achieve something, one thing that distinguishes those who go on to achieve and those who don't is mindset. If you can shift your mindset and realise that these are just excuses and make a concerted effort to flip these statements, you can achieve amazing positive change. Even something as simple as adding the word 'yet' or 'now' to the end of such statements can shift your mindset:

- I'm too busy *now*
- I'm too tired *now*
- I don't have enough money *yet*

You can then take this to the next level with statements such as:

- I'm too busy now, but I will get up 20 minutes earlier tomorrow and prepare a healthy lunch to take to work.
- I'm too tired now, but in the morning I will go for a 15-minute run.
- I don't have enough money yet, but I will transfer $50 a week to my savings account and by my birthday I can buy that shiny fancy thing I want.

Having a positive mindset is a big factor in developing positive habits. It's part of the desire component of the DARE model. You really need to have a growth mindset so you have an ability to look at your strengths and weaknesses and truly believe you are able to improve. A growth mindset enables you to believe you can change and believe you can achieve those changes.

Your desire, enthusiasm and commitment to achieve a goal will need to be at least a 7 or 8 out of 10 in order for it to be likely to succeed.

Accountability

Accountability is about making a commitment to taking certain action. It's easy to slip back into old ways if you are not being held accountable. You can achieve this by pairing up with another person, such as agreeing to go to the gym with a friend, checking in with your trainer, tracking your food intake on an app, or making an announcement to the world on social media. If someone else is aware of your desire to change, it is so much harder to fall off the wagon. The moment you make your goals known, you are more likely to stick to your game plan. There's nothing worse than telling people you are going to achieve something and never getting there. The pressure of a deadline is also powerful, such as entering a 5 km race in two months' time if you are new to running.

Here are some examples of being accountable:

- to another person – agreeing with a friend to go for a walk together at a certain time.
- to a group of people – telling your family and friends you are taking a break from alcohol.
- to the world at large – posting your commitment on social media that you will eat a healthy meal every day and posting a photo of the meal.
- to yourself – setting an alarm to go to bed by a certain time and sticking to it.

One of the things I did when COVID-19 first hit and gyms were closed was to devise my own at home training programs. But how could I make myself accountable in a lockdown? What I did was to place a tick on a calendar each time I did a workout. I like colour coding things, so I would place a big green tick on the days I worked out. On the days I didn't work out, I put a red cross. At the end of the month I had a clear visual representation of how many times I exercised. It can be quite revealing and also rewarding to see such a visual representation.

Reward

An important element of habit change is a reward. This helps to reinforce any positive change that you are attempting to achieve. Some changes take time to show any significant results so it is easy to get disheartened and feel like giving up. You may have been exercising and eating well for six weeks because you want to look healthy and strong, but you are not yet seeing any significant changes to your body, so you need small micro-rewards along the way to reinforce your positive habits and behaviour. One of the reasons why it can be difficult to stick with a positive habit, such as eating healthily or saving for retirement, is that it doesn't always give us an immediate reward, even though we know we can benefit in the long run. Therefore a good way to help make a positive habit stick is to find small rewards along the way to help reinforce the positive action you are taking.

Setting smaller goals can act as a reward and allows for more regular wins or rewards. For example, you want to run 5 km, but you are new to running. Break down the goal into smaller goals, such as "in one week from now I am running for 60 seconds at a time without stopping and in two weeks from now, I am running for two minutes at a time without stopping". These smaller goals help keep you motivated and act as mini rewards on the way to your larger goal of running 5 km.

Environment

While desire, accountability and reward are all critical, one of the most overlooked factors in endeavouring to create a new habit is the changes that you may need to make to your environment. This could be as simple as replacing all junk food in the house with healthy foods or even modifying who you interact with. But changing only your environment will not always lead to habit change.

> *"The key—if you want to build habits that last—is to join a group where the desired behaviour is the normal behaviour."*
>
> James Clear

Think about your behaviours and how much they are influenced by your surroundings and your connections. Do you drink too much on a Friday night because that's what your friends or colleagues do? Or do you get up early on a Saturday morning to go for a run with friends and grab a coffee afterwards because that is what that group of friends does? A deep human need for belonging can shape and influence our behaviours and our activities. So if you want to increase the likelihood of embedding positive habits, design your life and your surroundings in such a way as to make good habits easier and bad habits harder to follow. Find support for designing your environment by seeking out a tribe or community that supports those habits.

To help you apply the DARE Model in creating positive habits, I have developed a simple template that you can use:

My SMARTer lifestyle goal is…	
The SMARTer habit goal that supports my lifestyle goal is…	
My **Desire** for achieving this habit goal is…	
I will be **Accountable** by…	
I will **Reward** myself for doing this habit by…	
The changes I will make to my **Environment** are…	

Image 1b – DARE template

My story: part 1

I've discovered through trial and error that mindset is a critical component to positive habit change. Desire is a key part of the DARE Model and getting a habit to stick. If your heart is not really in to making the change, then it is unlikely to happen, despite all the good intentions, accountability systems and environmental changes that you make. A good example of this is when I wanted to go back to my music practice, or so I thought. I'd read a suggestion that if you want to play a musical instrument more, then put it in a place that is obvious. So for example, if you play the guitar, put the guitar in the living room where it is easily seen and is a visual prompt for you to pick it up and play it. So I adopted this idea and set up my electronic keyboard in my office right next to my desk. Hardly a day goes by when I am not sitting at my desk – working, checking emails or updating social media. How many times did I sit down at the keyboard and play? Next to never. Why? I couldn't understand it. It was right there in front of me every day. I had changed my environment to support a daily positive habit, but it wouldn't stick.

On reflection, I realised that two key elements of the DARE Model were missing. Firstly, accountability. I hadn't told anyone that this is what I was going to do. I hadn't committed to playing a piece of music for someone else (the pressure of the deadline!). Secondly, the desire wasn't there. I liked the idea of playing the keyboard more than the idea of seeing myself as a keyboard player. That is a significant shift in thought. You have to have the desire to have that habit be part of your identity, or you will not succeed. I didn't have that mindset, and to be honest, I am not sure that it is a priority in my life at the moment. Maybe in the future I will have a shift in thinking, but for now, the keyboard remains untouched. I have shifted my attention to implementing other habits that tick all four of the DARE boxes, building habits that are truer to me at this point of time in my life.

Is there anything else?

The DARE Model covers the basics of what you need to implement to create and embed positive habits in your life. But that is not always the whole picture. Your circumstances are likely to be unique and complex habits require more attention than easier habits. So, there are a range of other things that you can consider:

(a) Piggyback where you can – if you are already practising good habits, how can you utilise them and add another habit? For example, if you brush your teeth regularly but don't floss regularly, how can you piggyback off the existing habit of brushing your teeth to add flossing? One way I piggyback on existing habits is that I like to pick up groceries on my way home from the gym. I have to drive past the supermarket on my way home from the gym, and that is also the time of the day when I'm feeling energised and healthy, so I'm more inclined to select healthy foods when I go into the supermarket. In Chapter 2, there is an exercise that you can complete that will prompt you to identify any current habits that you can use to piggyback other positive habits.

(b) Parallel processing – are there things that you currently do automatically that would enable you to do something else at the same time? For example, when I used to work for a company that was in an area not well-serviced by public transport, I had to drive to work each day. I spent a lot of dead time in the car and the trip became second nature after a while. So I used the automation of that habit of driving each day to my advantage. I was studying at the time and I listened to my recorded lectures in the car, I listened to podcasts and audiobooks, and I would make a point of calling my parents every Wednesday afternoon on my drive home.

(c) Start small – only try to implement one or two habit changes at a time. If you try to change too much at once, you will spread yourself too thinly. We tend to overestimate how much we can do in a short period of time and underestimate what we can do in a long period of time. If something seems too hard or complex, then break it down into smaller steps. Don't be overambitious as that can lead to giving up and not reaching your goal.

(d) Good habits beget good habits – if you are able to embed one good habit, this can then be the foundation for introducing other good habits. For example, perhaps you have a goal of waking up half an hour earlier each day. Now that you are awake at an earlier time, you might go for a quick walk, prepare a homemade healthy lunch to take to work instead of buying takeaway, and you also end up saving money by making your own lunches. The one small change of waking up earlier has led to a number of other positive behaviour changes.

> *"Simplicity is the key to brilliance."*
> Bruce Lee

(e) Make small incremental change – you can't expect to harvest the fruit the day you plant the seed and you can't expect to complete a marathon until you have built up your running gradually. When I was in my twenties and thirties, I did some exercise but I was more of a bookish person. No one could have accused me at that time of being an athlete! But after my divorce at 37 years of age, I felt down and my self-confidence was low. I was looking for a positive outlet to help me feel better about myself. So I decided to take up running. I still remember the early days of going to the gym and shuffling along on the treadmill. I particularly remember the day I managed to run a whole kilometre in one go! I was so proud of myself. And I gradually added a bit more each time over the following months until one day I managed to run 10 km on the treadmill. Over the following twelve months I then started doing half marathons. This was in 2006. Fast forward to 2012 and I'm in the Sahara Desert with 120+ other people about to embark on my first ultramarathon. The event was a self-supported footrace of 250 km over seven days across sand dunes and rocky terrain in hot temperatures. Race organisers provided drinking water and tents to sleep in, but each person had to carry everything else they needed for that week, including food, first aid, a sleeping bag and change of clothing. It was the most amazing experience and it demonstrated to me that by incremental effort over time, I managed to achieve something that I never thought possible when I first started out on the treadmill in 2006. So, it's important to make small, simple changes gradually as this will help ensure that change can be long-lasting and sustainable.

"It's not what we do once in a while that shapes our lives. It's what we do consistently."
Anthony Robbins

(f) Consistency is more important than volume – just as is the case with incremental effort, being consistent, even if it is only a small amount at a time, will pay large dividends. Working out 20 minutes a day, six days a week, week after week, is more beneficial than doing a two-hour bootcamp once a month. Practising the piano for 20 minutes a day, every day, will yield better results than practising for one hour once a month. And you wouldn't brush your teeth 12 times in one day once a month; you brush your teeth 2-3 times a day, every day.

(g) Be kind to yourself – you will falter, that is the nature of any behavioural change, but persist. Think of a child learning to walk. They will fall over many times before they are up and stumbling around. When a child learns to walk and falls down 50 times, it doesn't think "I give up. This isn't for me." They keep going until they are finally able to walk. Also consider that if something is not working for you, it may not be the 'what' that needs to change, it may be the 'how'.

(h) Think about the language that you use – this feeds into your self-belief and desire. You may have a limiting belief and a simple shift in language can make a huge impact. For example, you may say to yourself that "I want to go the gym and do the HIIT class but I can't even do a push up". Simply reframing the statement by removing limiting words like "but" and adding the word "yet" can trigger a significant shift in your thinking. So the statement might instead be "I want to go the gym and do the HIIT class even though I can't do a push up yet".

Start with the simple DARE Model as your foundation to implement positive habits. As you start to form positive habits, consider whether you need to adjust or modify anything, such as piggybacking off other good habits or changing your self-talk.

My story: part 2

As a teenager and young adult I was a night owl. I would study until late and sleep in the next morning. Fast forward to today and I am now a morning person. What changed? When I was living in the Middle East and training for my triathlons and ultramarathons, it was usually too hot to train during the day. The coolest part of the day was the early morning before sunrise, so I would get my training done before work. There were many times when I would go for a two-hour run at 4.00 am or a three-hour bike ride at 4.30 am. I settled into the sleeping habit of rising early and also going to bed early. Even on the days when I wasn't training, I discovered that I could achieve a lot in those early hours of the day. Not many other people are awake at that time so you can get a lot done without being distracted or interrupted, which is more likely to happen towards the end of a working day.

I now find that I get a lot more done first thing in the morning rather than waiting until the evening. In the evenings, I tend to be mentally tired and less inclined to want to do things. For example, on the day that I'm writing this chapter, I have already been to the gym, been to the supermarket, checked and replied to emails, had breakfast, changed the bed and put out two loads of washing, made my next batch of kombucha, and written a few paragraphs of this book, and it's only just reached 9 am. I feel a sense of achievement, and I'm ready to tackle the rest of my day. The power of rising early has been recently documented in a number of books such as *The 5am Club* by Robin Sharma and numerous entrepreneurs and thought leaders such as Facebook's Sheryl Sandberg and Apple's Tim Cook are known for their early morning routines.

Aim for progress, not perfection

Can you be perfect all the time? No, and it is unrealistic to think you can be. So cut yourself some slack when you slip up. You can't go from being a couch potato to running a marathon in a matter of weeks. Taking small steps consistently over time is a key factor to success. Success is not always linear and there will be ups and downs. Failure is not the opposite of success. Failure is a stepping-stone on your way to success. Success is also about consistency, not volume. And when you do slip up – and you will – don't beat yourself up. And most importantly don't give up. A slip up is a learning opportunity. Reflect on why it happened and start anew tomorrow, and just keep going.

CHAPTER 2

Evaluate

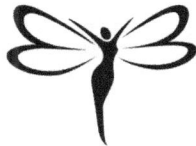

"You can't go back and change the beginning, but you can start where you are and change the ending."
CS Lewis

Introduction

What does your life currently look like? Do you find that you are busy with so many things but you feel like you are standing still or worse, going backwards? That you are unable to make progress with the things you want to change, such as eating healthier, exercising regularly, saving for your future, or reducing mindless time spent on social media?

You can't begin to make changes in your life if you don't know where you are now and you don't know where you are going. After completing this chapter, you will have:

1. Taken stock of your life.
2. A better understanding of your current reality.
3. A deeper knowledge of how you use your time.
4. Clarity around your goals and dreams.
5. Created a clear path for a better future.

This chapter will give you tools to help you take stock of your current situation and identify what you want your life to look like.

Where are you now?

There are various techniques you can use to assess your current situation. One of my favourite tools is a wheel of life[4], as this gives a strong visual representation of any current imbalances in your life. Balance is personal and unique to each individual. What may be satisfying for one person may be stressful or boring for another, so your wheel of life will be unique to you and can change over time.

The following wheel of life exercise is designed to raise your awareness about any imbalances in your life. It is the first step before planning a life that is more satisfying and can help clarify your priorities.

Be honest with yourself. If you can't be honest here in the privacy of reading this book and making your own notes that no one else will read, then you will never be honest with yourself!

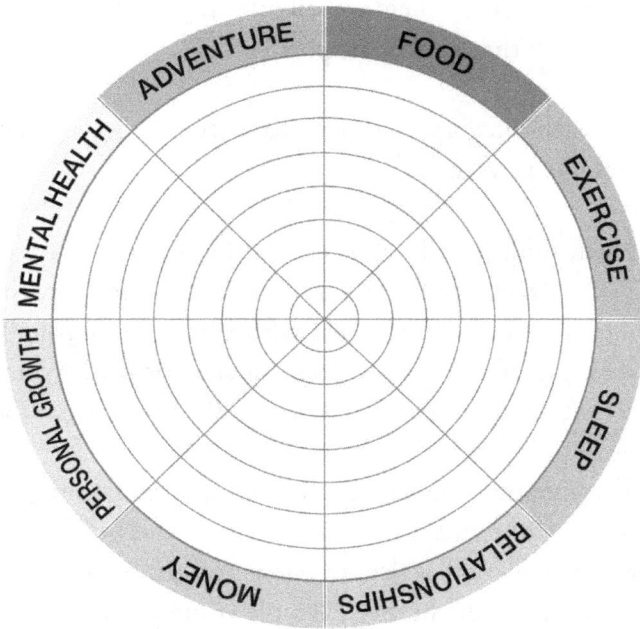

Image 2a – the wheel of life

Here's how to use the wheel of life:

1. Find a quiet space away from noises and distractions, turn off your phone, and think about the eight areas of your life as set out in the wheel of life.

2. The categories should together create a view of a balanced life for you. If you prefer, you can re-label an area to make it more meaningful for you. For example, replacing a category that is not relevant to you with a category that is, such as replacing 'money' with 'career'. Note that the categories set out in the wheel of life in image 2a are linked to specific chapters in this book, so if you substitute a category, then that new category may not be specifically addressed in this

book. However, there are still useful general tips throughout the book that may be helpful.

3. For each category, consider what success or satisfaction would feel like to you.

4. Next, rank your level of satisfaction with each part of your life by drawing a line across each segment to show the extent to which you are satisfied with that area of your life. For example, if you believe your satisfaction with your level of activity and exercise is a 4 out of 10, then draw a line at 4.

5. The lines that you have drawn should form an irregular shape in the circle and this is your current wheel of life. It should give you a good helicopter view of eight main areas of your life at the moment. See example at image 2b.

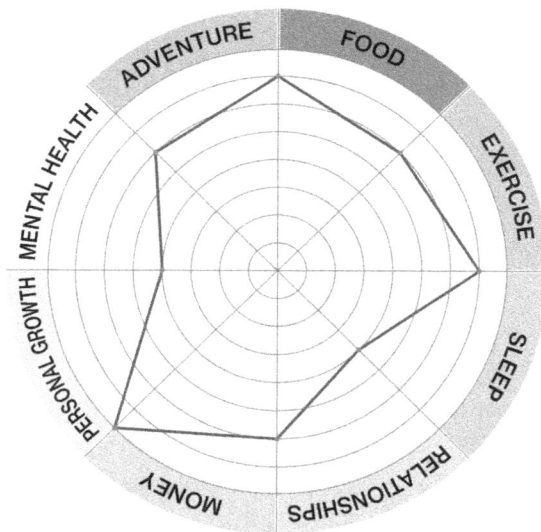

Image 2b – completed wheel of life example

Where are you going?

Before you can direct your life's journey onto a different path, you need to know where that path is going! In this section, we will drill down into what goals you want to reach.

In the completed wheel of life example in image 2b, you can see that the areas of money, food and exercise are ranked as being largely satisfactory, so the person in this example would probably not need to address these areas. However, the areas of personal growth, sleep and relationships rate quite poorly, so these are areas which may require more focus as areas of change.

What does your wheel of life look like and where do you want to go? Take a look at your wheel and ask yourself these questions:

(a) How do you feel about your life as you look at the wheel?
(b) Are there any surprises?
(c) How do you currently spend time in each of these areas?
(d) How would you like to spend time in each of these areas?
(e) What would a score of 10 in each area look like?
(f) Which of these areas would you most like to improve?
(g) How could you make space for making improvements in your life?
(h) What do you want to change first?

Devote enough time to reflect on these statements and think about what direction you want your life to take.

What are your goals?

Setting SMART goals

"Most people think they lack motivation when they really lack clarity."

James Clear

In Chapter 1 I touched on the notion that for goals to be effective, they need to be SMART. This means a goal has to be:

(a) **S**pecific – the goal needs to be clear and precise.
(b) **M**easurable – you need objective evidence to measure achievement of your goal.
(c) **A**chievable – a goal needs to be realistic and something you can reasonably be expected to accomplish, otherwise your motivation and belief can quickly disappear.
(d) **R**elevant – the goal needs to be relevant to you and to your values.
(e) **T**ime-based – a goal needs to have a target date for achievement for motivation and so you can also have a date to work towards.

How many times have you heard statements such as "I want to lose weight", or "I want to exercise more"? These sound like great goals, don't they? But they are not SMART goals. They may be relevant or achievable, but are they specific enough? Are you able to measure when you have achieved these goals? And by what time? If you are too vague with your goals, then you are less likely to achieve them.

Goals need to be measurable, otherwise you will have no idea whether you are making progress or not. Without some sense of progress, it is likely that you will lose motivation and momentum and you will be less likely to stay committed to your goal. For example, I recently took up weightlifting. In the beginning, I had no idea how to do a deadlift but I had a goal of lifting a certain weight by a certain time. I started out using minimal weight and, under the guidance of a coach, I improved my technique and slowly increased the weight I was able to lift. Over the subsequent months, I logged the repetitions and the weight I was able to lift each time I did a workout. The satisfaction of regularly hitting a new personal best every few weeks was incredibly rewarding! After many months of consistent training, I am now able to easily deadlift considerably more than my body weight. Being able to measure and easily quantify my progress has been a huge factor in me continuing to improve and get stronger and fitter each day.

How achievable is your goal? It needs to be a goal that you can achieve over time. For example, setting a goal such as "I will never eat chips again" is unrealistic and puts too much stress and expectation on you every time you go shopping or dine out. You are setting yourself up for failure.

I would also add a sixth element to the SMART goal model. The goal should be positively expressed. So for example, rather than saying you want to lose weight, express it in a more positive way, such as reaching a target weight instead. A SMARTer goal should also be expressed in a way as if it has already happened.

SMARTer goals would be:

"It is 30 September 2021, and I weigh 72 kg."

"It is 31 October 2021, and I am walking for 30 minutes a day, four times a week."

Make a distinction between a lifestyle goal and a habit goal. A lifestyle goal is a desired outcome. A habit goal relates to the regular practices you need to undertake that will support your lifestyle goal. An example of a lifestyle goal may be to reach a certain weight by a certain date. An example of a habit goal that would support your lifestyle goal may be that you will eat six healthy serves of vegetables a day.

So, based on your wheel of life assessment, what are your SMARTer lifestyle goals?

Happiness versus pleasure

Before we look at what your SMARTer lifestyle goals could be, ask yourself, what makes you happy? Is this something that you have given any thought to? Many people when asked this question will measure their happiness by some external factor, for example, owning a nice car or binge-watching Netflix. But is that really what happiness is?

Happiness is a feeling of contentment and fulfillment, an element of life satisfaction. Happiness is a more stable state and it should not be confused with pleasure or joy, which are more transient, short-lived and in the moment. Pleasure often refers to sensory-based feelings we get from experiences like eating good food, getting a massage, receiving a compliment, or having sex.[5] There is nothing wrong with experiencing pleasure and in my view we should all endeavour to seek pleasure in our lives. But pleasure should not come at the cost of happiness, for example, seeking pleasure and comfort in food or alcohol, which can then undermine our health goals and our ultimate happiness.

Daily decisions

Did you know we make more than 35,000 decisions every day?[6] This number may sound absurd, but in fact, we make more than

36

220 decisions each day on just food alone according to researchers at Cornell University.[7] Sounds incredible, doesn't it? One observation from that study is that many food-related decisions occur in distracting environments and may lead to mindless eating.

Think about the decisions you make each day in relation to food. What about those unconscious actions you take, particularly if you are distracted? Do you eat your meals while scrolling on social media or watching tv? Are you really paying attention to what you are eating and if you have reached satiety?

Many of the decisions we make each day are subconscious, from the words we use (and we use an average of 16,000 words a day) to driving a motor vehicle.

With this in mind, you can see how easy it is to continue with unhealthy habits. But on the flipside, it can also be used to your advantage; to set up healthy habits as part of your daily decision making.

What habits do you currently have?

Do you have a daily routine? What does it look like? Is it the same as yesterday, last week, or even last year? Having a routine suggests being rigid or inflexible, but in fact it creates a whole new open space for you to be creative by automating your habits.

The creation of positive, sustainable habits will not only benefit you in the long run by improving your overall quality of life, they can also help you maintain positive patterns when life throws you a curveball.

In the next exercise, the goal is to identify what habits you currently have that you could potentially 'piggyback' off. For example, you may brush your teeth twice a day – after breakfast and after dinner. You have a goal of getting fitter. You could then, for example, use your teeth brushing as a trigger to build an additional habit of doing 20 push-ups and 20 sit-ups after you brush your teeth. Or eating lunch as a trigger for going for a 10-minute walk afterwards. The idea here is to use any existing habits as a platform to build additional positive habits into your day that are aligned with your goals.

Image 2c is a table that will help you identify any daily habits that you currently have, such as brushing your teeth, driving to work, making your morning coffee, taking a shower, walking the dog, and so on. This is a brainstorming exercise, so don't spend too much time analysing or judging these! The goal here is to simply identify what your current regular habits are. Spend about 15-20 minutes brainstorming this, with no self-editing or filtering.

Current habits	Frequency
Walk the dog	Daily every morning
Brush teeth	Twice a day after breakfast and dinner
Morning coffee	Daily every morning
Drive to/from work	Daily on weekdays
Go to the bathroom	6-7 times a day
Shower	Daily
Drop off/pick up kids from school	Twice a day on weekdays
Music lessons	Once a week

Do the laundry	2-3 times a week
Change the bed linen	Weekly
Soccer practice	Weekly
Apply make-up	Daily every morning

Image 2c – habits brainstorming checklist sample

The next step is to then look at those habits and identify the ones that you believe can be used as the basis for adding on an additional habit. In each lifestyle chapter – Chapters 4 to 11 – you will have an opportunity to drill down and think about what positive habits you can introduce into your life.

Regular reviews

Apart from establishing lifestyle habits – such as eating healthier or exercising more – you should also consider setting up the habit of undertaking a regular evaluation of your life. As humans, we are not static; we evolve, grow and change, and over time, our goals can also change. That's why it is useful to do a regular audit of where you are in life and where you want to be going. I do this on an annual basis and the start of each new year is when I reflect on the past year and visualise what the coming year could look like. But you may decide to do an evaluation more frequently or less frequently, or at another time of the year.

Here are some ideas that may prompt you to come up with your own evaluation plan:

1. In the first week of a new year, undertake a review of where you are and where you want to be. You can use the wheel of life as a tool to evaluate your life.

2. Create a vision board and at the start of each year consider if it is still true to your goals.

3. Use a large year planner whiteboard to map out your year ahead. I use mine to plan my races and sports goals for the year ahead using colour coding, for example, I write up my key races in red and secondary races in blue. I also use it to block out any other commitments, for example, career training days which I write up with a green marker.

4. Conduct an annual review at the time you have to submit your annual tax return (or when you have to submit quarterly payments).

5. Use your birthday (or any other anniversary) as a time to reflect on and evaluate your life.

Creating space

Eliminating things from your life can be challenging. What is forbidden often becomes more appealing simply because we can't have it or can't have as much of it as we want. Think of certain foods as an example. If the major portion of a meal was dessert, rather than a healthy entrée, you would probably find yourself craving more of the entrée. Now reverse the situation where you have an abundance of healthy food but choose not to eat dessert. It can be easy to feel like we are missing out if we decide to never eat ice cream again, for example. But this often leads to making that eliminated food more appealing and after time, you are likely to binge on it. The key message here is that sometimes completely removing something from your life is not the answer, unless it clearly no longer serves you and is not in line with your values. Sometimes reducing or modifying is enough to make a positive shift in your life.

In the next chapter, we will look at ways that you can remove or reduce things from your life to create space for positive change.

CHAPTER 3

Delete

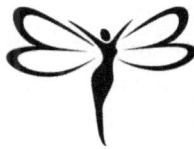

"As you remove things from life you don't need, you find more time for the things you do."

Joshua Becker

Introduction

Our lives are so busy, with many of us rushing from one task to the next and often we feel overwhelmed as a result. Everyone around us also seems so busy and there never feels like there are enough hours in a day. How do you then add new things to your life when it is already so full and busy? One approach, and arguably the most achievable and sensible one, is to remove things that do not serve you and do not support your goals and dreams.

If you are serious about making positive changes in your life, then you need to create space in your life for that change. There are only 24 hours in a day – and we all have the same number of hours – but some of us use those hours more wisely than others. Creating space will reduce your stress and brain clutter, result in peace of mind and open up an opportunity to become a better version of you. It can also lead to increased happiness, greater enjoyment of life, improved fulfilment and heightened success.

How to create space

So why are some people better than others at getting things done? One key to success is prioritising and creating space for the things that matter. Does your day start with checking emails, doing small chores and tasks and responding to other people's demands? If so, then the chances are that you are not doing the things that really matter to you. It's easy to fill our time with trivial tasks but then we are often left wondering where our day, week or month went. Focus on the big stuff, the things that matter, and you will always find a way to get the smaller things done.

Many people say they are too busy and there are not enough hours in the day, but it is usually a case of how you are using those 24 hours that we all have.

Look to remove things from your life that don't support you and your long-term goals. For example, is binge-watching Netflix enriching your life? Does going to after work drinks every Friday support your health and weight loss goal? Ultimately, we are not too busy, we just choose to give priority to some things over others. We have the power of choice.

Before you start to think that I am suggesting you remove all joy from your life, I'm not! What I am suggesting though is that there may be areas of your life that are not serving you and I am asking you, where are you spending too many hours? Are you binge-watching Netflix for four hours a night? Are you scrolling through social media for three hours every day? That's 21-28 hours a week, or 45-60 days a year! Binge-watching Netflix for four hours a day every day equals two months of your year. Just let that sink in for a minute. That is two whole months of a year, or 16% of your life. Are you therefore that busy not to fit in other things in your life?

Consider whether these types of activities support you in being the best version of you. You don't have to eliminate these activities but consider reducing them. So instead of spending four hours binge-watching Netflix, consider watching only one hour and using the other three hours on something you have always wanted to do but keep putting off because you are 'too busy', such as going to the gym or doing meal preparation. I admit it, I have binge-watched shows, and it was great! I loved it. But I have been judicious in the time I spend doing this. I haven't then compromised on other areas of my life that are important to me, such as eating well, getting quality sleep and exercising.

The same goes for the scenario of going to after work drinks every Friday. Rather than doing this every week, consider reducing this to only once a fortnight, and use that time to instead go to the gym, meal prep or engage in an activity that supports your goals.

Use technology as your friend. For example, there are numerous apps and features on our devices that can monitor our time spent on them. If you have a smart phone it will tell you how much screen time you use each day and week.

The flipside is that technology can improve the quality of our life in so many ways and can make us more efficient and productive. Technology has given us a number of benefits. For example, to watch live or catch-up commercial television now, you don't even need a television. If you have a smart device like a tablet or smartphone, you can stream live television on those devices. The same goes for streaming services like Netflix, Stan and Amazon Prime. Unfortunately, this also allows these technologies to intrude into other parts of our lives. One benefit though is that such devices are portable so you can then catch up on shows while doing other activities such as commuting. I am a big fan of listening to podcasts and audiobooks during so called 'dead' time, such as when I am driving or catching the train or bus.

As I mentioned, you don't need to completely remove things from your life but think about how you can better prioritise your time.

What things are most important to you and how do you create space for them? Go back to your wheel of life exercise in Chapter 2 and see where your priorities are.

My story

Let me share some of my stories with you that may encourage you to make similar changes in your life.

I regularly check my emails first thing in the morning. Some time ago, it occurred to me that my inbox in the morning had more than 50 emails, mostly stuff I had subscribed to a long time ago, but that I don't bother reading any more. I bulk selected and deleted most of these emails every morning. While it didn't take much time to do this every day, that time does add up, and there was also the mental toll of having to decide every day which emails to send straight to the bin. I had only been awake for half an hour and yet I was already mentally tired. Not a great way to start each and every day. So what would you do in this situation? You may do what I ended up doing. One day I didn't delete those emails but I set aside time later that afternoon to go through them one by one. I then ruthlessly unsubscribed from all but the most relevant ones. I wasn't reading most of those emails anyway, so I unsubscribed from 90% of them. Over the course of the following week, I repeated the exercise. While it took an upfront investment in time to unsubscribe from various emails, it now means I start each day reading emails I actually want to read and not bulk deleting them without even looking at them.

Another example of when I was able to better prioritise my time was when I was training for long-distance triathlons and ultramarathons. If you are not sure what a long-distance triathlon or ultramarathon is, then let me break it down for you. A long-distance triathlon involves a 3.8 km swim, followed by a 180 km cycle, and finishes with a marathon – a 42.2 km run. You must complete the event in under 16 hours. As for the ultramarathons I have done, they have been self-supported multi-day staged events across some of the toughest terrain in the world, such as the Sahara and Gobi Deserts. This involved running a set distance each day, totalling 250 km over seven days. Over those seven days, you have to carry all your food, your sleeping bag, clothes, first aid and any other essentials in a backpack. The only things that race organisers supply are drinking water and tents to sleep in. As you can imagine, you don't take on these events lightly. If you want to finish a long-distance triathlon or an ultramarathon, you have to train and you have to be prepared. Each event involved at least six months of serious training. So when I was preparing for those events, my life was essentially train, eat and sleep. I still found time to socialise and have fun, but I addressed things like excessive watching of tv shows and cut back on this type of activity as it didn't support my overall goal of completing a triathlon or ultramarathon. I also made a point of socialising on only 1-2 nights a week. Additionally, I told my friends – my amazing support crew – what I was doing and why I was doing it so they understood and supported me. So while I didn't eliminate certain things from my life like watching my favourite shows or catching up with friends, I was more selective and structured in how I used my time so I could meet my ultimate goal.

Ideas

Is your life now as you want it? Probably not if you are reading this book. You will have to make tough decisions on what things stay in your life and what things don't. This does not need to be permanent, as you can always adjust as you go or simply reduce rather than remove things from your life altogether.

Here are some ideas that I have discovered or that others have shared with me that may prompt some changes in your life and reduce all those unnecessary burdens on your time:

1. Delete apps off your smart phone, tablet etc. and use the web-based versions of apps such as Facebook and Messenger, or at least turn off the notifications for apps or turn off mobile data. This includes not just social media, but also emails and messages. Choose the time that you wish to read these messages rather than being reactive. If something is super urgent someone will call you or find another way to reach you. You don't need to be checking your messages 50 times or 100 times a day.

2. Hide the television remote or its batteries to make it harder to fritter away hours in front of the television.

3. Block out time in your diary for activities and stick to it so that your time doesn't drift. For example, if you are going to lunch, commit to leaving at a certain time.

4. Unsubscribe from mailing lists – be ruthless!

5. Consider outsourcing tasks that you don't believe add value to your life, such as housework, gardening, or admin such as bookkeeping or social media. If you run your own business, you could consider hiring a personal assistant to do social media, bookkeeping and other tasks for a set amount of time (for example five hours a week) to free up your time and your headspace to pursue more valuable tasks.

6. Some people simplify their environment to be almost Spartan in nature, with no television or other modern comforts. This may suit you, but I am of the view that this may not be sustainable for everyone, particularly from a mental health point of view, as we all need a bit of lightness and joy in our lives.

7. Look at each activity you do each day and honestly ask if that activity is taking you closer to your goals or not.

8. Set specific times of the day to go on social media and set an alarm to get off social media.

Digital detox as an example of creating space

We spend so much of our time on our phones, tablets, computers or other technological devices that are meant to make our lives simpler and easier. But you know what? Our lives are now busier and more distracted than ever. I came to the realisation some time ago that I was spending a lot of time on my devices and going down various internet rabbit holes, and then realising that I was just squandering large chunks of my day. And then I would wonder why I couldn't get things done. So I decided to do a digital detox and you know what I discovered? By reducing my time on my devices and being more targeted in my consumption of social media, I was able to free up eight hours a week. That's a full working day for most people! What can you achieve in eight hours? What other things can you find time for if you reduce your time spent in other areas?

To undertake a digital detox, start by identifying the type and amount of consumption of media, especially social media. Most devices these days can give you a breakdown of the amount of time you spent on each platform. You might be surprised at the hours that you spend per week on Facebook, TikTok or other apps.

Then look at what amount of that time is essential (for example, you may use social media to promote your business) and how much of that time is optional (think playing online games and watching TikTok dance videos).

The next step is to decide what your goal is. If you are currently spending 20 hours a week on your devices, with ten of those hours being essential (for example, posts related to your business) and the remaining ten hours being optional, then you may want to reduce your optional digital consumption time by five hours a week. That's around 45 minutes a day, which is not a large amount of time, but enough to free up space for you to do more meaningful things, such as reading a few chapters of a book or preparing a healthy dinner instead of ordering delivery.

So your SMARTer goal may look like this: "It is 30 June 2022 and the time I spend on optional digital media consumption is no more than five hours a week".

Applying the DARE Model

So how could you apply the DARE Model? It could look like this:

My SMARTer lifestyle goal is…	It is 30 June 2022 and the time I spend on optional digital media consumption is no more than five hours a week.
The SMARTer habit goal that supports my lifestyle goal is…	I will check social media at predetermined times only – at 8.00 am and at 5.30 pm on weekdays and at 10.00 am on weekends – for only 15 minutes at a time.
My **Desire** for achieving this habit goal is…	8 out of 10.
I will be **Accountable** by…	Letting family and friends know that I will be selective and targeted with my time on social media.
I will **Reward** myself for doing this habit by…	Using the time that I would otherwise be on social media to instead prepare quick and healthy meals.

The changes I will make to my **Environment** are...	Turn off notifications on my phone and tablet for all social media and emails.
	Block out 15-minute 'appointments' in my calendar on my phone at 8.00 am and at 5.30 pm on weekdays and at 10.00 am on weekends to check social media.
	Block out 20 minutes of time once a week to go through my emails and unsubscribe from unnecessary mailing lists.
	Charge my phone and tablet outside of the bedroom so I am not tempted to scroll through social media before bed and when I wake up.

CHAPTER 4

Rest

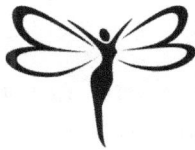

"Sleep is the best meditation."

Dalai Lama

Introduction

Do you often find you get your best ideas when you are in the shower, when you are driving, or when you are swimming, walking or dreaming? You are not alone! The brain needs regular breaks, so rest and quality sleep are necessary elements of how our body functions. We tend to be more creative too when we are at rest, when we are relaxing or when we are alone. Sleep is the most powerful form of rest and many of us do not get the minimum amount of quality sleep each night. Getting enough good quality sleep is seriously undervalued, as it impacts so many aspects of our life.

Health impacts of poor sleep

Some people believe that they can function well on only a little sleep, boasting that they only need five or six hours a night. They proudly proclaim, "I can sleep when I'm dead!" What they probably don't realise though, is that lack of sleep will most likely send them to an early grave, and they are at higher risk of developing metabolic diseases such as obesity, stroke and type 2 diabetes.

So what happens to our bodies when we don't get enough sleep and what is the connection with modern diseases such as those mentioned above?

When we don't get enough sleep, our cortisol levels rise. Increased levels of cortisol in the body can trigger an increase in cravings for carbohydrates, particularly sugary foods and this then sends our glucose levels up, which in turn can trigger weight gain, particularly an increase in belly fat, and puts us at higher risk of developing type 2 diabetes. Various studies have shown that people who sleep less than seven hours a day are at significantly higher risk of developing type 2 diabetes and obesity.

One study found that getting insufficient sleep can cause changes in more than 700 genes and has adverse impacts on your body.[8] Even one night of poor sleep can result in lower creativity[9] and an increase in anxiety and stress.

A lack of sleep can also adversely impact your microbiome. Our microbiome has been recognised as an organ in its own right and is a community of beneficial microbes, mainly in the gut, but also elsewhere such as in the mouth and on our skin. The microbes in our gut aid our digestion by helping us absorb nutrients from food, regulate our immune system and even produce vitamins such as vitamin B12 and vitamin K. We have only just started to explore the microbiome and understand the importance of it to human health. However, a lack of sleep has been shown to increase the bacteria in our microbiome which then is able to extract more calories from the food we consume as it passes through our digestive tract, which can lead to weight gain.

Numerous studies also link sleep deprivation with eating more calories (particularly from processed foods) and weight gain. Other research indicates that sleep deprivation can increase cravings for high carbohydrate foods, especially foods that are calorie-dense such as chips, bread, and biscuits. It is believed that sleep deprivation influences two of the hormones in our body – leptin and ghrelin. Leptin is the hormone that is responsible for signalling that we are full and ghrelin signals when we are hungry.

What is the right amount of sleep?

Most people are at their peak if they get between seven and nine hours sleep a night. Apart from the health benefits of getting enough sleep, getting seven to nine hours of sleep a night will give you more energy throughout the day and ensure you are more alert and focussed. Studies have shown that driving while sleep-deprived is equivalent to having had a few alcoholic drinks, with your responsiveness and alertness being significantly reduced and your decision-making being adversely impacted. Driving when you have had fewer than six hours sleep can triple your risk of having a car accident. Other consequences of not getting enough sleep include exhaustion, brain fog, heart conditions, reduced sex drive, and irritability.

Leptin increases naturally during the day and peaks in the evening while ghrelin levels increase just before food intake, suggesting that ghrelin rises and falls in line with our normal meal routine. However, if you stay awake and are sleep-deprived, this can negatively impact these hormones. A University of Chicago study saw an 18% decrease in levels of leptin and a 28% increase in levels of ghrelin in subjects who were sleep-deprived.[10] Another effect of sleep deprivation is that we are more likely to make poor choices when we are tired. When we are well-rested, we are unlikely to eat a whole packet of Tim Tams, but at 12.30 am, this may seem like a good idea.

A number of people take the approach that they don't need to sleep during the week and they will make up for it on the weekend. However, as with many things in life, consistency is key. Sleep deprivation for the majority of the time cannot be overcome by sleeping in on the weekend. Your body has its own natural circadian rhythms.

Circadian rhythms

Circadian rhythms are 24-hour cycles that are essentially your body's internal clock. Arguably the most important of these would be the sleep-wake cycle, and exposure to light is a significant factor that triggers this cycle. Generally our strongest desire for sleep is between midnight and 6.00 am, however, in our modern world, we are exposed to light at times when our natural circadian rhythm should be entering the sleep phase. Watching movies late at night and using our mobile phones or other light-emitting devices before bed can contribute to the disruption of our sleep cycle. New parents, people who work shifts or work late or early, or who travel across time zones regularly, are likely to have disrupted or poor-quality sleep. Visually impaired people who have no perception of light can also experience a disruption to their circadian sleep rhythm as they do not receive light information.[9] People living in polar regions can also have their circadian rhythms adversely affected by the long, dark winters and almost 24 hours of daylight in summer. People in northern Europe have reported incidents of midwinter insomnia.[11] According to Professor Josephine Arendt, "The lack of natural bright light during the polar winter means that the main time cue for the organization of circadian rhythms is greatly diminished". Similarly, during the 24 hours of daylight, the circadian rhythms are disrupted. Carefully timed light exposure in winter and the use of eye masks or block out blinds or curtains in summer are some of the approaches people in these regions use to support the body's natural circadian rhythms.

What about pills?

Did you know that bright light from mobile phones, tablets, computers, and televisions blocks the release of the sleep hormone, melatonin, after only 1.5 hours of using technology in the evening? Melatonin is a hormone that is critical for controlling the body's day and night cycles. The human body produces melatonin and more is released when it is dark to help a person fall asleep. If the production or release of melatonin is blocked or reduced, it can cause sleep problems and can also exacerbate mental health issues such as depression.

Taking melatonin as an oral supplement may be a short-term fix to re-set the body clock (for example after prolonged sleep issues or because of jet lag), but it is not a long-term solution and you should speak to your medical professional before taking any melatonin supplements.

Some people also rely on sleeping pills to overcome sleeping issues, but this is also only a short-term fix and should only be considered as a last resort and in consultation with your medical professional. Sleeping pills are addictive and you build intolerance to them over time, so with prolonged use you need more and more to get the same outcome, which is dangerous. Taking sleeping pills also doesn't address the underlying problem of why you are not getting quality sleep.

Sleep cycles

It's not just the duration of sleep that is important – the quality of sleep you get is also critical.

Our sleep goes in cycles, alternating between light sleep, deep sleep and REM (rapid eye movement) sleep. In the light sleep phase, you are more likely to wake up easily. The deep sleep phase is necessary for you to feel rested when you wake up and if you wake up during this sleep phase, you are more likely to feel groggy and unrested. The REM sleep phase is characterised by your eyes moving behind your eyelids and is the phase where you dream.

Deep sleep is important as this is when your body repairs any damaged tissue. REM sleep is thought to be the time when your memories are consolidated and helps learning and improved mood.[12] Research suggests that a lack of REM sleep can reduce your coping mechanisms, increase your likelihood of getting migraine headaches and is associated with an increase in weight.

How do you know if you are sleep-deprived?

Here are some signs that you may be sleep-deprived and not getting enough quality sleep:

- You are tired and irritable
- You wake up a lot during the night – disrupted sleep probably means that you are not reaching stages of deep sleep
- Increased appetite
- Weight gain, especially around the belly
- Frequent yawning during the day
- Daytime fatigue

- Difficulty concentrating and focussing on tasks
- Poor memory
- Looking fatigued – dark circles under eyes, saggy or puffy eyelids, pale or dull skin
- Reduced sex drive

Objections

When I speak to people about making sleep a priority, these are some of the main objections I hear:

"I'm a night owl. I don't get tired until late."

That may be true, but if you are regularly burning the midnight oil and do not wake up feeling refreshed, then something is amiss. Try unwinding before bed with something calming such as a warm shower, a cup of non-stimulating herbal tea (such as chamomile or valerian tea) and try going to bed 15 minutes or 30 minutes earlier than usual. Gradually adjust over time. Alternatively, try rising later in the morning and prepare all the things you need the night before such as prepping breakfast, putting out your gym and work clothes, and making your lunch.

"I have too much to do before bed."

Is it the end of the world if some chores wait for another day? Do you really have so many urgent things that can't wait a day or two or even a week? You will always have things to do. Use your time wisely. Sleep is probably more important than doing the ironing, filing paperwork, or scrolling through social media. Make sleep a priority. Tasks or chores that really are not urgent can wait for another day.

Ideas

Here are some other ideas that may help you get better quality sleep:

1. Use technology to set an alarm for bedtimes and waking times, and to monitor your sleep. An app like Sleep Cycle can be helpful to identify sleep cycles, sleep duration, and even if you snore! Some apps also use music and delta waves to induce sleep, such as BrainWave.

2. Set a daily reminder on your phone that tells you to turn your phone off or to put it in flight mode at a certain time, for example, 9.00 pm every night, or use a filter to block out blue light and reduce the brightness of your phone. Most devices now have a night-time setting that adjusts the colour of the display to warmer colours.

3. Invest in a good mattress and comfortable pillows and replace them regularly (mattresses should be replaced every 8-10 years and pillows every 12 months). Also invest in the best quality bed linen you can afford. You spend roughly a third of your life sleeping, so why not make it a comfortable experience! I love hotel beds with king size mattresses and crisp high quality bed linen and I try to recreate that feeling of comfort in my own home.

4. Consider using scented candles (but don't fall asleep with a lit candle!) or an oil diffuser with calming oils such as lavender or chamomile.

5. Avoid alcohol and food (especially rich or heavy food) in the 2-3 hours before bed. When you eat, your digestive system is

active and as a result your core temperature is raised. If you avoid eating in the few hours before bed, this can help keep your body's core temperature down, which can help trigger sleepiness.

6. Mentally (and if possible, physically) close the kitchen and the bar at a certain time in the evening. For example, I live in an open plan home, so there is no door to the kitchen, but I mentally close the kitchen around 7.30 pm after cleaning up the dinner dishes. This is also an example of piggybacking off another habit – cleaning up the dishes after dinner is the trigger for mentally closing the kitchen.

7. Avoid coffee, tea, cola and other caffeinated drinks after lunch. Caffeine has a half-life of 12 hours which means 50% of that midday coffee is still in your system 12 hours later.

8. Your bedroom should be for sleep and sex only. Remove anything that may cause noise, such as your mobile phone, and could wake you from your sleep and remove other devices such as a television, laptop and tablet. At the very least, put your phone and other devices in flight mode at night. If you do use your mobile phone as your alarm, then create a physical distance between yourself and technology in the bedroom, for example, put your phone on the other side of the room and not near your head.

9. Where possible aim to be exposed to natural light first thing in the morning. Take your cup of coffee outside, do some stretches or yoga on your balcony or in the backyard, or go for a walk around the block before breakfast. Exposure to sunlight increases your body's production of serotonin. Serotonin regulates a number of bodily functions, including

mood, appetite and sleep. Only 15-20 minutes of exposure to natural light first thing in the morning, every morning, can contribute to better quality sleep.

10. Eat a healthy diet. Serotonin is mainly made in your gut and a healthy diet will influence its production, which can lead to improved sleep.

11. Change light globes from a blue light to a warm light in the bedroom and in other rooms where you use artificial light before you go to bed. Warm colours, particularly red, have been shown to be conducive to sleep. Also ensure they are a low wattage or lower in lumens (a measure of the level of brightness), as softer lighting will also be more conducive to sleep.

12. Have a hot bath or shower an hour before bed and then cool down. The body's core temperature will drop and help you relax and go to sleep.

13. Keep your bedroom temperature at around 17 degrees Celsius if possible.

14. Do some quiet activity in the evening, like meditation, listening to soothing music or stretching.

15. In the hour or two before bed, start dimming lights in the house.

16. Sleep in total darkness if you can. Block out curtains or eye masks are some options to consider.

17. 'Dump' any thoughts and mental chatter by writing these down before you go to bed. This can help reduce or eliminate any mental chatter that can keep you awake at night.

18. If you have trouble falling asleep, consider doing some deep breathing exercises before bed.

If you find that you are still struggling with your sleep despite trying these or other tips, consult your medical professional. In Australia, it is estimated that 10% of Australians suffer from undiagnosed sleep apnoea.[13] Sleep apnoea is a chronic health condition where your breathing may be limited, or you may stop breathing, in your sleep. Symptoms include restlessness and waking up during the night, feeling constantly fatigued, and snoring. Speak to your medical professional for more information and for advice.

Applying the DARE Model

Applying the DARE Model could then look like this:

My SMARTer lifestyle goal is…	It is 3 April 2022 and I am getting at least 7 ½ hours of quality sleep a night.
The SMARTer habit goal that supports my lifestyle goal is…	I will be in bed by 10.00 pm on weeknights and by 11.30 pm on weekends.
My **Desire** for achieving this habit goal is…	8/10.
I will be **Accountable** by…	Telling my spouse, children and friends about my goal and why it is important to me. Using a sleep app to monitor my sleep and to track my sleep statistics.
I will **Reward** myself for doing this habit by…	Buying silk pillowcases when I achieve my habit goal consistently after two weeks and I will buy new sheets when I continue to achieve my habit goal after six weeks.
The changes I will make to my **Environment** are…	Change light globe in bedroom to warm light. Remove the tv from the bedroom. Remove phone chargers from the bedroom.

CHAPTER 5

Nourish

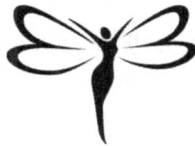

"Fuelling your body with nutritious food is the highest form of self-respect."

Unknown

Introduction

When people say to me that they want to eat healthier food, I will ask them, what is your why? Is it to lose weight? Is it to feel better? Is it to change body composition? Or do you have a different motivation? You need to be clear on your why. As mentioned in Chapters 1 and 2, the first part of the DARE Model is being clear on your desire for change and setting a SMARTer goal is critical. Why do you want to eat healthier food?

Benefits of healthier food choices

In 2017, two in three Australian adults were overweight or obese, which is interesting, as Australia is often perceived as being a fit and healthy nation. Data from the Australian Bureau of Statistics show that Australians generally have a poor diet, that we do not eat enough fruit and vegetables and that we eat too many discretionary foods that are high in salt, fat and sugar. Fewer than 10% of the population meet the recommended intake of 5-6 serves of vegetables a day.[14]

Some of the benefits of eating more nutritious and healthy food are:

(a) Having more energy – eating nutrient-dense food that is not calorie-dense will provide your body with 'cleaner' energy. Think about the circumstances where you might want more energy, such as playing with your children or grandchildren.

(b) Overall health – eating better will assist in fat loss and there is a saying that 'abs are made in the kitchen'. In other words, nutrition is key for fat loss. You are also more likely to get all the vitamins and minerals you need to support your body's functions and its immune system.

(c) Reduced risk of disease – eating well can help reduce the risk of metabolic diseases that are related to lifestyle choices, such as type 2 diabetes, heart disease, obesity, stroke, and even some cancers.

(d) External appearance – eating more 'clean' foods such as fruits and vegetables and drinking more water will improve the appearance of your skin, hair, nails and eyes. Poor diet often means that you will look older than you really are.

(e) Mental health – ongoing research has indicated that there is a strong connection between the brain and the gut microbiome. Eating healthier has been shown to contribute to improved mood, lower anxiety, better memory, less brain fog, and improved self-confidence.

(f) Better sleep quality – some foods, such as fish, fruit and vegetables show sleep-promoting effects. There is growing evidence that indicates sufficient nutrient consumption is important for sleep and that a lack of key nutrients, such as calcium, magnesium, and vitamins A, C, D, E, and K are associated with sleep problems.[15]

(g) Better body composition – exercise as much as you want, but if you want to lose weight or change your body composition by reducing your body fat, the most significant factor is your diet.

By the way, I really do not like the word 'diet'. It suggests some restrictive form of eating and some level of misery. It doesn't need to be that way. Diet is really about what foods and drinks you choose to put into your body. My philosophy is simple. It essentially boils down to maximising nutrients while not consuming excessive calories.

Weight loss and body composition

If your focus is on losing weight then, unless you are viewed as seriously overweight or obese, you may want to consider shifting your thinking to instead make your goal to change your body composition. In simple terms, your body fat takes up more space in your body than muscle. Muscle is denser than fat and will occupy less space than fat. I am not a fan of scales but prefer to use a measuring tape and a body composition scale (which you can find in places like gyms and nutritionist's offices) which will give you an assessment of how much muscle and body fat you have.

Due to a running injury, I recently stopped running and was looking for something else to do to keep fit. I settled on weightlifting. I had several goals, such as the amount of weight I would be able to deadlift after six months and what my body composition would be after that time. Over the course of those six months, my weight on the scales barely changed but my waist and hip measurements declined by a few centimetres, my body fat percentage decreased and my lean muscle increased. Weightlifting was part of the story, but I was also eating a lot more cleanly and tracking what I was eating. The message here is – be clear on your why and what your goals are and use meaningful measures to assess whether or not you are reaching them. Weight loss may not necessarily be the appropriate goal for you. Consider whether you should instead focus on reducing the percentage of body fat or find another meaningful goal such as reducing your waist circumference. A high waist circumference (more than 94 centimetres for men and more than 80 centimetres for women)[16] is linked to an increased risk of chronic disease such as type 2 diabetes, heart disease and sleep apnoea.

If you are obese, then speak to your health professional. Obesity over time will catch up with you and can lead to a number one killer – heart disease. There is also a correlation with high blood pressure, high cholesterol and diabetes, and it is a comorbidity to many other conditions.

What about BMI?

BMI stands for 'Body Mass Index' and is calculated by dividing your weight in kilograms by your height in metres squared. So for example if you weigh 70 kg and are 170 cm tall the formula is $70 \div (1.7\text{x}1.7) =$ 24.2. A BMI of between 18.5 and 25 is considered to be in the healthy range while a BMI of more than 30 is considered to be obese. There are flaws with BMI as a measure of health as it doesn't take into account that muscle is denser than fat, so fit body builders and high-performance athletes can have a high BMI purely because they have a high level of muscle. It is also flawed when used with others in the general population, such as pregnant women.

Feeling better

There is increasing evidence to support the notion that the quality of the food you eat not only influences your physical health but can also improve your mental performance. Just like a car, your brain functions best when it gets premium fuel. Fuelling your body with high-quality foods that contain lots of vitamins and minerals nourishes the brain. Eating clean and introducing more vegetables and fruits can improve digestion and waste elimination, make you feel more energised and improve your mood. There is also increasing knowledge around the importance of the microbiome and its impact on mental health. Recent studies have demonstrated the positive influence of a healthy microbiome on patients suffering from anxiety and depression and how gut inflammation can impair mental health.[17]

"Knowledge is power."
Francis Bacon

Macros and calories

The second element of the DARE Model is to be accountable. One way to do that which I find is helpful for many people, including myself, is to track your macros each day.

Macros (or more correctly, macronutrients) are the three main nutrients we need in significant amounts to survive. They are protein, carbohydrates and fat.

Micronutrients are nutrients that we need in smaller amounts, such as vitamins and minerals.

The amount of energy in our food is measured in units of energy called calories. The average, moderately active adult needs about 2,000 calories (for women) to 2,500 calories (for men) a day.

There are a number of diets that are promoted as the be all and end all to fat loss and weight loss. But they all essentially work off a similar premise – energy in versus energy out – and dieting approaches such as intermittent fasting, keto, or vegan tend to work (at least in the short term) as they all ultimately will reduce the number of calories you consume by restricting the amount of food or types of certain foods that you eat.

My food philosophy is to keep it simple, make it sustainable, and make it enjoyable! I believe that achieving and maintaining a healthy weight essentially comes down to energy in versus energy out, so I recommend you keep track of your calories and macros (at least for the short-term) to help you better understand what energy you are consuming.

There are many apps out there that are easy to use such as MyFitnessPal where you can enter your target calories and macros per day and then enter the foods and drinks that you consume each day. You can also keep a bound paper food diary, which is a great visual way to see what you consume each day and helps with accountability. What the macro breakdown is will vary from person to person and again there are numerous websites and groups on social media that can assist here (see for example Macros Inc), or you can seek the services of a professional such as a nutritionist or personal trainer. I have a personal trainer who not only sets my weightlifting program, but also cycles my macros depending on the phase of my training, such as muscle gain or maintenance. Currently, I am on 1,850 calories a day with 28% of those calories coming from protein, 40% coming from carbs, and 32% coming from fat. This split of macros is tailored particularly for me, taking into account my activity level, age and the training stage I am in.

It is important to understand that those percentages do not relate to the physical weight of those macros, but the energy – that is, the calories in those macros. So a gram of carbohydrates has four calories, a gram of protein also has four calories while a gram of fat has nine calories. Note that alcohol has seven calories per gram but has no real nutritional value.

If you consume 150 calories more per meal than you actually need, that's an extra 450 calories per day if you eat three meals a day. That adds up to an extra 3,150 calories per week. How does this impact your body? Well, the body tends to store any excess calories as fat. 3,500 calories equates to half a kilo of fat. So if you overconsume even just 100 calories a meal for 12 days, you could gain up to half a kilo in fat. If you do that for 120 days that's five kilos, and after a year, that's 15 kilos. So you can see how easy it can be for your weight to slowly creep up.

What does 100 calories look like? It's one slice of bread. Or ½ a cup of cooked rice. It's 14 almonds. It's a third of an avocado. None of these foods are unhealthy. They can form part of a healthy diet. But the key message here is portion size and to be knowledgeable about your food.

If you track your food for at least a few weeks, you will have a greater awareness of what calories and macros you are consuming which will help you make better food choices.

Some people believe that they must starve themselves to lose weight, but that is actually counterproductive. Your body needs a certain level of calories each day to function properly. See Chapter 8 – Move and the section on understanding how your body uses energy.

The importance of protein

I recommend that you include some form of protein in every meal, even breakfast, and this could be as simple as adding yogurt to your cereal or adding a scrambled egg to your toast. Protein is more satiating than carbohydrates, as it takes longer to digest and can leave you feeling fuller for longer. Our modern western diets also mean that many of us do not get enough protein per day. Going back to my macro breakdown, 28% of my calories should be coming from protein, which is about 130 grams a day on a 1,850 calorie diet. It is also important to understand the makeup of the food you are eating, as a 200-gram chicken breast is not the same as 200 grams of protein. A 200-gram chicken breast will have about 62 grams of protein. If you are vegetarian or vegan, it is even more critical to consider tracking your macros as plants are not as significant a source of protein as meat. Vegetables that are high in protein include edamame (11 grams of protein per 100 grams) and chickpeas (8.4 grams of protein per 100 grams). Brown wheat flour has around 12 grams of protein per 100 grams and nuts are high in protein, but are also high in fat, which can significantly increase your calorie intake, so be aware the next time you reach for a nutbar or a handful of nuts.

What about fat and sugar?

We are currently living in a highly toxic food environment, an environment of very palatable foods that are heavily processed and that keep us addicted and interested in those foods. Unfortunately, more often than not, they also deliver a large number of calories without much nutritional value and without always making us feel full.

One of the biggest issues with a modern western diet is that we consume a large amount of sugar, usually through eating prepared foods such as salad dressings, prepared pasta sauces, and even foods that are touted as healthy, such as low-fat yoghurt and low-fat ice cream. Foods where the fat is removed or reduced will taste bland as a result, as fat is a carrier for flavour, so food manufacturers tend to replace the fat with sugar to make the food more palatable. Look at the label of any processed food, even something like a jar of pasta sauce, a tin of baked beans or a readymade salad dressing. The ingredients of those foods will generally be listed on the label in descending order by weight, and sugar tends to be high up on the list. Next time you do your grocery shopping, set aside some extra time to read the ingredients list on the labels of processed food before you purchase anything and you may be surprised how much sugar there is in the foods we eat.

Sugar, in particular fructose, is pervasive in many of the foods we consume. Fructose is found in fruit, but it is also found in high fructose corn syrup (which is found in many commercially made foods such as sodas and even pasta sauces) and table sugar. So should you eat less fruit? Current studies indicate that our biggest source of fructose intake is from sugar-sweetened beverages like Coke and Fanta (30%), followed by grains (22%) and then actual fruit (19%). On that basis, we should perhaps focus on reducing our sugar intake from commercially available foods such as sodas and processed foods. It is important to also consider that commercially produced foods do not provide the additional nutrients such as fibre, vitamins, and minerals that fruit provides.

As for low-fat foods, I am not a fan because:

(a) we do need some fat in our diet. Fat is important for hormone regulation and for the absorption of certain vitamins such as vitamins A and D. I get my dietary fat from meat, oily fish like salmon, olive oil and butter, nuts and dairy, including cheese, yoghurt and eggs, and from avocados.

(b) fat is a carrier for flavour, and to make low-fat food taste more palatable, manufacturers will often add a lot of sugar. Consumption of sugar releases endorphins and dopamine, and dopamine disables our ability to act logically, as it turns off our logical pre-frontal cortex thinking. Repeated consumption of such foods increases dopamine levels over time and as we build up a tolerance, our dopamine receptor levels reduce, and as a result we require more sugar to experience the same level of satisfaction and pleasure.

(c) it can give a false belief that it is healthier or lower in calories than a full-fat version, but this is not always the case. A simple example is comparing full cream ice cream with a low-fat ice cream. Many brands of low-fat ice cream add more sugar to make the ice cream more palatable and therefore the calorie count for low-fat versus full cream ice cream may not be that different.

"Eat food, not too much, mostly plants."
Michael Pollan

Simple and sustainable

The average human adult eats almost 700 kg of food in a year. That is bound to have a serious impact on your body, particularly if you are not eating mostly nutritious food. You are what you eat. So is it garbage in, garbage out? Or are you nurturing your body? For me, my principle is that I take care of my body and care about what foods I put into it. It is not so much about the length of my life, but the quality of my life. More and more, I see people around my age who have mobility issues due to being overweight. I still want to be independently mobile and able to be active into my older years, and not rely on a mobility scooter or be confined to my home simply because my weight or poor health prevents me from living a full life.

Improving your nutrition and eating healthier foods isn't complicated. Preparing and eating food should be enjoyable and eating healthier should be something that can easily fit in to your lifestyle.

Some people get caught up worrying about whether they should have one egg or two on their morning toast, or one or two teaspoons of olive oil on their salad, but then don't think twice about having three glasses of wine with dinner or two large scoops of ice cream in the evening. Don't get too caught up in the small details and take a broader perspective. I tend to aim for 80-90% of my nutrition being on point, which allows for the occasional 'fun food' such as a glass or two of wine. Get it mostly right and you'll find you will feel more energised and your mood will lift.

I am also not a fan of diets or lifestyles that eliminate certain foods or whole food groups (unless of course you are allergic to those foods or you do not consume them as that is part of your faith). Eliminating your favourite foods will make you sad and you are likely to just end up bingeing on them later. If you have a favourite treat, you don't need to eliminate it altogether, but explore ways that you can reduce your intake, especially if the food item has high calories but little or no nutritional value. Chocolate and alcohol are good examples of such foods as they are high in calories but don't offer much in the way of micronutrients. Have a clear understanding about the difference between a food being calorie-dense and nutrient-dense. An apple may have 100 calories but is rich in fibre, vitamin C, potassium and phytonutrients such as quercetin and chlorogenic acid, both of which are antioxidants. Compare this with four small squares of milk chocolate (about 17 grams), which is also around 100 calories, but is high in saturated fat and offers little to no nutritional value. Other chocolate treats don't do much better with half a Snickers bar, 2 Kit Kat fingers, 1 ½ Lindor balls and half a 35-gram Freddo Frog all having 100 calories each. As you can see, it can be relatively easy to overconsume calories with your favourite treats, and these portions are unlikely to make you feel full or give you the nutritional benefits of an apple.

There's also a reason we're often told to eat more fibre. Fibre is not only good for your digestion, but it also takes time to digest and will make you feel fuller for longer. So for example, apples are high in fibre which will be slower to digest than a glass of apple juice. Eating an apple instead of drinking apple juice will also prevent an insulin spike with a burst of energy, followed by the drop in energy immediately after. Eating whole foods is beneficial in levelling out your sugar levels and also stabilising your mood, minimising those hangry moments.

Vitamin supplements

What about vitamin supplements? While they may have a place if your diet is not in order, if you are eating a healthy and nutritious diet, then you probably don't need them. Real foods will usually contain all the nutrients you need such as vitamins, minerals, fibre, and phytonutrients. Rather than spending money on supplements, spend it on healthy and nutritious whole foods. The only exception I would make here is that due to the mass production of many of our fruits and vegetables, the soils in which such foods are grown may be depleted, so the update of important minerals may be compromised. Also, the length of time some produce takes to get from farm to plate can see a diminishing in nutrients by the time you put that food in your mouth. If you are concerned, speak to your doctor about doing some blood tests to see if you are deficient in any vitamins or minerals. And don't assume. Here are some stories of my experiences with deficiencies.

My story

I lived in the Middle East for 10 years and I assumed that since I was in a part of the world that had sunny days for most of the year, my vitamin D intake was sufficient (one way we get vitamin D is that it is produced by your body in response to exposure to sunlight). Unfortunately, that was not the case for me or for many others who I knew in that part of the world as we did spend many hours inside, particularly in summer, in air-conditioned comfort while it was 50 degrees outside. I essentially addressed this by spending at least 20 minutes outside in the early morning to get my vitamin D hit.

Another example is when I was training for and competing in a 50 km ultramarathon in the beautiful Blue Mountains in Australia a few years ago. It was a tough race, with more than 2,400 metres of elevation gain but I struggled a lot more than I had expected. I felt nauseous, fatigued and spacy during training sessions and during the race. I started well but gradually fatigued and fell further and further back in the field. I fumbled to the finish line in a less than impressive time, felt plain awful and I don't remember too much about finishing. I knew something wasn't right. I felt off but I didn't know why. Fast forward to a few weeks later when I was getting my blood work results from my doctor and he told me I had extraordinarily low iron levels. This was a shock to me as I thought my diet was balanced and on point. Various investigative procedures later (including a colonoscopy and endoscopy – ugh!) failed to show any serious cause for the low iron levels. That was a huge relief, but it was a reminder to me that I need to be more tuned in to what I am eating and track what I eat. That was a huge turning point and while I was on iron supplements for a while, I no longer need them or take them.

"If you fail to plan, you are planning to fail."
Benjamin Franklin

Meal planning

Meal planning for me is all about doing as much preparation as possible when you have available time. Generally, we don't have a lot of time on weeknights, particularly if we've had a long day at work. If we are also tired, we are more likely to also make unhealthy food choices. I'm a big advocate of cooking your own food as you then know exactly what goes into it. Often food in restaurants will be much higher in calories than home-cooked meals. A large portion of the time that goes in to cooking your own meals is usually the preparation, not the cooking itself. Activities such as peeling and chopping vegetables, crumbing schnitzel, or washing and preparing salad ingredients take time. Instead, use an hour on a Sunday to think about the week ahead and prepare some of your meals in advance. This does not have to mean making ten portions of spaghetti Bolognese! The idea of eating the same meal for five or more days in a row may suit some people, but it doesn't fill me with joy. Meal prep on a Sunday can be as simple as chopping vegetables that you are going to roast on the Tuesday and popping them into a Ziplock bag with some herbs and olive oil, or washing, drying and chopping salad ingredients and separately shaking up a salad dressing in a jar with a lid that you can keep in the fridge. I prefer to prep my own salad ingredients as it is more economical than the pre-packaged bags you get in the supermarket, plus, I'm sure you've experienced the frustration of opening a bag of supermarket salad greens that are wet and a bit slimy. Yuk! As for salad dressing, I make my own because (a) it's easy as there are only a few ingredients, and (b) the prepared dressings you find in the supermarkets tend to be high in sugar.

I know some people object to meal prep because they believe it is too time-consuming or they have tried it before and it hasn't worked for them. My response is that I find if I utilise my environment to support me by blocking out time in my week to do it, it gets done. I find the small investment upfront on a Sunday pays out huge dividends in the ensuing week by saving me time in making dinner, especially when I am tired. It also ensures that I am more likely to make smart food choices during the week.

I have to admit that I did struggle in the beginning to get into the habit of preparing the foundations of my meals once a week, so I had to reassess and find out why I was struggling. The simple answer was I had started out on a day and at a time that didn't fit in with my social habits. So I tweaked my routine and tried a different approach. I am now in the habit of regularly planning my meals in advance. It was not the 'what' that was the issue, but the 'how'. I also called on my support network and made sure I was accountable (for example, via social media) to help me achieve my goals. And the reward was knowing each week my dinners were healthy, easy to prepare and the mental burden of knowing what to make was significantly reduced. Don't forget, the process is about progress, not perfection. Every beginning will be challenging but the long-term rewards are worth it.

Also don't underestimate the power of leftovers. One of my favourite ways to meal plan is to do a roast on a Sunday night, usually a roast chicken with a range of roasted vegetables such as potatoes, pumpkin, sweet potato, carrots, and with a side of steamed green vegetables such as beans, asparagus or zucchini. I always make more so that I can use leftovers in the following days. This doesn't mean eating the same meal for 3-4 days in a row but being creative with the leftovers. For example, leftovers from a Sunday roast of chicken and vegetables can mean a chicken and salad sandwich for lunch on Monday, a chicken and roast pumpkin risotto on Tuesday (with the cooked chicken bones used to make the stock for the risotto) and a chicken and roast vegetable salad with a pesto dressing on Wednesday. These aren't difficult or fancy meals, but they are healthy, economical and easy to prepare as well as offering a bit of variety.

Meal planning or meal prepping also helps reduce wastage. Recent research has shown that 53% of Australian households throw out food from their fridge at least once a week, which results in close to $4,000 of groceries per household going to waste every year. This also contributes a shocking 7.3 million tonnes of food waste annually. Further research indicates that 30% of Australians want to be more organised in the kitchen and 37% are trying to reduce their food waste.

Planning your fridge and pantry can be as important as planning your meals. Who hasn't stood in front of a fully stocked fridge and said, "I don't know what to make"? I have been guilty of this! One way to reduce the mental burden of deciding what to cook is to organise your fridge based on meals rather than ingredients. For example, group milk, yoghurt and berries together for breakfast, and group chicken, Asian green vegetables and Thai curry paste together for a dinner idea. It is then much easier for you to visualise a meal and it can reduce the mental toll of deciding what to make.

If you are a novice cook or if you are not a confident cook, find five meals that are delicious, nutritious, quick and easy to make and learn how to make them well. You will then always have something on standby to make if you have to work late or if you are otherwise short on time. Bookstores are overflowing with cookbooks nowadays and looking on websites and in bookstores for cookbooks and recipes for inspiration can be overwhelming. Meanwhile, television shows like MasterChef Australia are inspiring and make for great food porn but can place a lot of pressure on people to produce extraordinary meals using molecular gastronomy and fancy techniques. Do we actually cook such dishes in our own home on a Wednesday night after an exhausting day at work? Unlikely. Think of the meals that you enjoy the most. For me, simplest meals are always the best – particularly midweek – using good quality ingredients. I love cuisines such as Italian and Asian, as they place importance on the quality of the produce with minimal ingredients.

But I just don't like vegetables and fruit!

I hear this from many people. For whatever reason, they generally just don't like vegetables and fruit, or don't like particular vegetables or fruit.

The first thing you should ask yourself is, why? Why don't you like these foods? Is it the texture? The taste? A bad experience growing up when vegetables were boiled to death and were grey, tasteless and unappetising?

If any of these are true, then think about how to prepare these foods in a different way. For example, I am not a fan of boiled brussels sprouts. But roast them in an oven and serve them with bits of crispy bacon, toasted hazelnuts, a squeeze of lemon juice and a drizzle of olive oil, and they are delicious.

One of the worst food crimes is overcooking your vegetables. Quite frankly, there is nothing worse than soggy, overboiled vegetables. In my opinion, cooked vegetables such as beans, carrots and asparagus should be still 'to the bite' and slightly firm in the middle with some resistance when you bite on them. If you are still not convinced that vegetables can be delicious, consider also cooking them in a different way. For example, I like to cook carrots in a saucepan with some butter and herbs such as parsley, thyme or tarragon, or roast them in the oven, instead of boiling or steaming them.

As for fruit, we are incredibly lucky in Australia that we have such wonderful produce all year round. I especially look forward to summer as that is when juicy peaches, plump cherries and my favourite, amazing mangoes, arrive. If you don't like fruit, then again ask yourself why? Is it the flavour or texture? Is it something else? Sometimes a bad experience can put us off from trying the same thing again. I recommend that you spend some time in your local fruit and veg shop and see the abundance of produce available. Whenever possible, I always try new things. It has meant I have discovered the exquisite taste and texture of the mangosteen and the delicate flavour of the persimmon. I also love berries, in particular blueberries, raspberries and blackberries, and I will happily eat them straight from the punnet. Not only are they full of nutrients, but they are delicious and filling due to the significant amount of fibre in these fruits. If you are struggling to eat fruits, think of ways to gently introduce them to your diet, for example, having a serve of berries with a small scoop of good quality vanilla ice cream for a simple dessert.

Eating out

What if your work means that you regularly attend functions, dinners and events? This makes it challenging to make healthy food choices and it would be unrealistic and unsustainable to restrict such events. Therefore factoring in such events in your overall weekly meal planning can assist you in making better choices outside of those events. My philosophy is to aim to be healthy 80-90% of the time. And when you have a treat, don't feel guilty about it. Enjoy it, knowing that you are eating well most of the time. Another way to look at it is if you eat 35 meals a week (breakfast, lunch, dinner and two snacks a day) then this means that around 30 of your meals each week should be healthy. Another approach is to have healthy snacks or light meals such as a salad on standby that you can have before an event and then you are less likely to overeat and overindulge at the event. Ultimately, planning is key.

Shift your mindset

It is also important to aim for a mindset of nourishing your body, not depriving it. Over time, you will find it easier to have a mindset of making choices that are good for you, particularly if you are prone to reaching for comfort food and tend towards emotional eating. Emotional eating is not a grumble in the stomach. Emotional hunger and emotional eating can be caused by any number of other factors. As the name suggests, this type of hunger is not physiological, but has an emotional or psychological trigger.[18] The most common are boredom, stress and to fill an emotional void. Emotional hunger will usually result in craving specific comfort foods and can lead to unhealthy choices such as eating a whole large pizza or a large tub of ice cream by yourself. My basic test of whether my hunger is physiological or emotional is, if I am really hungry, I will happily eat an apple. Try this trick next time you want to binge eat on some sugary treats after dinner. If you are concerned that your eating is triggered by emotional needs, seek out the support and advice of a health professional.

Another mindset consideration is to think of any dietary adjustments as just that. They are adjustments, not deprivation or elimination. Adopt a mindset of modification not restriction and think of ways to implement this in practice. For example, rather than having a slice of cheesecake for dessert, share it with your dining companion, so you can still enjoy it, but you have reduced the portion you are consuming. Another example is if you regularly go out for a burger with friends on the weekend. Rather than avoiding the socialising, consider modifying your meal to have the mini burger rather than the large burger, or get a smaller portion of chips, or share the chips with your dining companions.

What about alcohol?

In 2019, Australians spent an average of $1,621 on household consumption of alcohol. In 2020, the year of the COVID-19 pandemic, there was a considerable increase in spending on alcohol, with Australians spending an average of $1,891 in that year.[19]

If we go back a few years before the pandemic, there are some even more staggering figures. In 2016, Australians spent $1.6 billion on tea and coffee, $12.6 billion on meat, and a whopping $14.9 billion on alcohol.[20]

Ironically, the expenditure on alcohol per capita is more than double the cost of your average gym membership.

Many people enjoy an alcoholic drink but there has been a shift in Australia where the number of ex-drinkers is on the rise, with weight gain and hangovers being the main reason for people giving up alcohol. Many people are 'sober curious', meaning they are keen to reduce or stop their alcohol consumption, bring a questioning mindset to a drinking situation and challenge the dominant drinking culture.

Alcohol consumption is sold as a glamorous event by marketers – think of all the ads that show happy people celebrating a birthday, a birth, or a wedding with a glass of alcohol – but the reality is somewhat different. Alcohol is one of the highest risk factors contributing to the burden of disease in Australia[21] and in 2018-19, 36% of drug treatment episodes were primarily for alcohol, making it the most commonly treated drug in Australia. Apart from the increased risk of preventable disease (for example, there is a correlation between alcohol consumption and an increased risk of breast cancer in women)[22], alcohol contains no nutritional value but a lot of calories.

Many people are also not aware of what a standard serving size is. In Australia, a standard alcoholic drink is a drink containing 10 grams of pure alcohol. Servings of alcohol in pubs and clubs are often higher than what is considered a standard serving. A standard glass of red wine is 100 ml (while a pub serve may be 150 ml) and a large glass of full-strength beer (about 425 ml) is 1.6 standard drinks.

I am not saying you shouldn't drink alcohol – I enjoy an occasional glass of red wine – but if you do drink, then perhaps reflect on your behaviours and ask yourself if there is scope to reduce your current consumption. Assess how much you currently consume and see if you can reduce it by say, 25%. Or take a week or a month off, for example by supporting charities such as FebFast and Dry July. If you take a break from alcohol, you may notice that your sleep improves, your skin looks clearer, and you wake up feeling fresher and more energised. And if you choose to drink, take it into account when looking at your calorie intake and macro intake.

Ideas

Some ideas that you may want to consider are:

(a) Liquid calories can add up quickly, so ditch the sports drinks when you work out and drink water. Unless you are exercising for more than an hour or in very hot conditions and are perspiring excessively, you don't need to consume sports drinks. Water is all you need. Similarly, soft drinks and sodas can quickly add to your calorie intake. Be aware that sugar-free options are not necessarily a smart choice. Studies have shown that people who routinely use artificial sweeteners may start to find less intensely sweet foods, such as fruit, less appealing and unsweet foods, such as vegetables, unpalatable. Several observational studies have also found that using artificial sweeteners and drinking high amounts of diet soda is associated with an increased risk of obesity and metabolic syndrome. Consider too whether your three caffé lattes a day or two glasses of wine are adding empty calories (three caffé lattes can be as much as 400 calories and two glasses of red wine can be 300 calories or more).

(b) Start your dinner with a garden salad with dressing or a small vegetable-based soup and you are less likely to overeat when it comes to your main meal. I sometimes like to start my evening meal with a salad as an entrée. Sounds odd I know. But I do this for two reasons. Firstly, it is a great way to get extra vegetables into my diet. Secondly it is filling enough (thanks to the vegetables being high in water and fibre) so that by the time I eat my main meal, I am less inclined to overeat as I already have food in my stomach. Stretching out my meal like this is a great way to utilise the fact that it takes about 20 minutes for your brain to register that your stomach is full. As a bonus, the salad will be low in calories, but high in water and fibre, and is an example of food that has a low calorie density. Calorie density is a measure of the calorie content of a food item relative to the weight of that item. Foods that are low in calorie density will make you feel fuller with fewer calories as they tend to have a higher water or fibre content, such as fresh vegetables and fruit. I aim to eat at least 25-30 different fruits and vegetables a week, and vegetables or fruit at every meal. This not only ensures a diversity of micronutrients but my gut microbiome loves it too.

(c) Fill your plate with vegetables. My general rule of thumb is 50% vegetables, 30% protein and 20% starchy carbohydrates. So an example might be a garden salad of mixed salad vegetables that fills 50% of my plate, a portion of fish that fills 30% and roasted potatoes that fill 20% (or you could have another carbohydrate such as pasta or rice). Another option is to sneak vegetables into meat-based dishes, such as Bolognese sauce, by adding finely chopped vegetables such as mushrooms, carrots and zucchini.

(d) Do you have chocolate cravings? This may actually be a sign of magnesium deficiency. Many people are deficient in magnesium and it is a mineral that is vital for proper functioning of your body. Talk to your health care professional about whether you should take a low dose magnesium supplement. If you are able to supplement with magnesium, take it before bedtime as magnesium can make you sleepy and don't take too much as this can lead to gut-related issues such as diarrhoea and nausea.

(e) If you are planning a night out at a restaurant, take a look at the menu on the restaurant's website before you go and decide what you will eat. When you are at the restaurant, don't be afraid to order first. Research shows that we are often influenced and swayed by what other people order when we dine out. So if others order first, you may be tempted to follow suit and not stick to your plan.

(f) Be mindful of sauces and condiments such as mayonnaise, aioli and other calorie-rich options. Yes, they are tasty and have a place in the enjoyment of food, but by simply omitting these from your meal you can save up to 200 calories per serve.

(g) Do you find that you crave sweet things in the evening? Something as simple as switching the timing of brushing your teeth in the evening can make a difference. For example, don't wait until before you go to bed to brush your teeth. Immediately after dinner, brush your teeth. You may find that your sweet cravings diminish. Other people find success with chewing a stick of gum if they have a sweet craving in the evening.

(h) During a busy work week, I like cooking meals that don't require a lot of hands-on attention. For example, I like to make meals that are as simple as roasting vegetables and some chicken, or meals that can sit on the stovetop without you having to constantly monitor them. This frees up time to do other things in parallel, such as catch up on emails or spend some quality time with your family.

(i) Invest time for meal prep and stick to it. Block out time on a day when you are not that busy (such as a Sunday afternoon) to do some basic preparation of ingredients and meals for the week ahead.

(j) Set a daily calendar alert on your phone or other device to do certain things, such as track calories, track macros, drink water, set the table for dinner and so on.

(k) Review your pantry and clear out foods and restock. If you struggle with overconsuming certain high calorie, low nutrient foods such as chips, chocolate and wine, then make access to them harder. Either remove them, don't purchase them or put them in hard-to-reach places.

(l) Do you shop based on 'feel'? Or based on a well-formulated plan? I prefer to plan as I am then not tempted to buy other things – those shiny new things in supermarket aisles that are marketed to us but that are not necessarily good for us – and I stick to the plan. Some of the tactics I employ to support me in this are having a magnetic paper-based shopping list on the fridge that I can quickly and easily add to when I am in the kitchen if I will be doing a physical visit and shop at the supermarket, or prepopulating my online shopping basket with my food choices on my favourite online supermarket websites.

(m) When you are shopping at a supermarket, do you notice that the real food is around the perimeter and the highly processed food is in the centre aisles? So, the next time you go grocery shopping, go around the perimeter as much as you can as this is usually where the fruit, vegetables, meat, seafood and dairy are situated and you are then more likely to make healthier food choices.

(n) Eat more protein. When you eat, it actually temporarily speeds up your metabolism thanks to what is known as the Thermic Effect of Food (TEF). This is because your body burns calories to be able to digest food. Protein increases your metabolic rate by 15–30%, compared to 5–10% for carbohydrates and 3% for fats. See also Chapter 8 – Move.

(o) Learn some basic knife skills. This not only allows you to show off to your family and friends, but it will literally slice time off your food prep time. Invest in some good quality knives too. This may seem expensive but they will stay with you forever if you look after them and they will probably outlive you. If you are on a budget, at least invest in a decent chef's knife, a bread knife and a paring knife. Having good quality knives will seriously improve your cooking experience.

(p) Get better quality sleep. Various studies link lack of sleep to obesity and if you are not getting enough sleep, chances are you are storing fat. A lack of sleep increases ghrelin (the hormone that makes you feel hungry) and decreases or blocks leptin, which is the hormone that tells you that you are full after eating. See Chapter 4 – Rest.

(q) Don't shop on an empty stomach. Studies show that we make poorer food choices at the supermarket when we are hungry. Instead, plan your shopping with a list and go at a time when you know you won't be hungry, such as after dinner. Or order online and be judicious in your food choices.

(r) Identify triggers that can help you get in the habit of consuming more water. Hunger pangs can instead be a sign that you are actually dehydrated, and I have also discovered in myself that if I feel tired in the afternoons or I am experiencing brain fog, it's usually because I haven't had enough water that day. Your test for knowing if you are drinking enough water is the colour of your urine. If it is a pale straw colour, then you are properly hydrated. If you don't like drinking water because you believe it is dull and flavourless, look for ways to jazz it up. Some options are using a SodaStream or similar device to carbonate your water, drinking from a fancy glass rather than a plastic sports bottle, or using fruit, vegetables or herbs in your water such as strawberries, cucumber slices or mint. You could even pre-freeze pieces of fruit and herbs with water in ice cube trays. I love sparking water. I am happy to drink it plain, but sometimes I will add some lemon or mint. I usually drink 2-3 litres of water a day, sometimes more if I am engaging in strenuous exercise or if the weather is particularly hot and I am perspiring more than usual. Hydrating well is an important component of your overall nutrition. If you are dehydrated you are more likely to feel tired, have muddled thinking and feel foggy, be constipated, have mood fluctuations and have low energy. Being dehydrated can also give you false hunger signals, meaning you are more likely to reach for a snack instead of a glass of water. Also our bodies, particularly our joints, require hydration to function properly. Don't use disliking water as an excuse not to stay hydrated. Experiment with different ways to make it more enjoyable for you.

(s) Carry healthy snacks with you. If you have healthy snacks on hand, you are less likely to be tempted to make an unhealthy food choice if you are hungry and not at home.

(t) Consider using the services of a meal delivery company such as Hello Fresh or Marley Spoon. These can be helpful as they minimise food wastage and are generally nutritionally balanced meals, with lots of vegetables. But check the calorie content of meals when you are ordering.

The bottom line

So what's the bottom line? My principles of healthy eating are fairly simple and can be summarised as follows:

(a) Eat more vegetables, especially leafy greens and non-starchy vegetables.

(b) Eat protein at every meal.

(c) Eat foods closest to their natural state as possible.

(d) Drink more water. I always start and end my day with a glass of water and I always have a bottle of water next to my bed and on my office desk.

(e) Track your macros and calories so you understand portion sizes and how much energy (i.e. calories) you are consuming each day.

Applying the DARE Model

So how can we use the DARE Model to create heathy eating habits? Here is an example:

My SMARTer lifestyle goal is…	It is 2 August 2022 and I am eating six healthy serves of vegetables and fruit a day.
The SMARTer habit goal that supports my lifestyle goal is…	I will have at least two serves of vegetables or fruit at every meal.
My **Desire** for achieving this habit goal is…	9/10.
I will be **Accountable** by…	Posting photos of my meals on Instagram. Using an app to track my food which my personal trainer can access and see.
I will **Reward** myself for doing this habit by…	Buying a new Nutribullet when I achieve my habit goal after two weeks and I will buy new gym leggings when I continue to achieve my habit goal after six weeks.
The changes I will make to my **Environment** are…	Remove all junk food from the pantry and fridge so I am not tempted to eat it. Prepare vegetables on Sunday so they will be ready to cook when I come home from work in the evenings during the week. Reorganise the fridge so that fresh vegetables and fruit are at eye level when I open the fridge door.

CHAPTER 6

Stretch

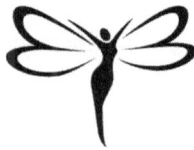

"A ship is safe in a harbour, but that is not what ships are built for."

John Shedd

Introduction

When is the last time that you did something that was exhilarating or that put you outside of your comfort zone? Do you remember the feeling you had? Were you apprehensive beforehand but afterwards glad that you pushed yourself? As humans we sometimes let fear dominate our lives. Fear of failure. Fear of pain. Fear of the unknown.

But what if we were to try anyway? Anyone who knows me will know that one of my favourite sayings before attempting something new is "What is the worst thing that can happen?" And usually nothing bad does happen. I go on to have an amazing experience and wonder why on earth I was worried or hesitant in the first place.

> *"If you never fail, you're only trying things that are too easy and playing far below your level."*
>
> Eliezer Yudkowsky

Getting out of your comfort zone

Why should you get out of your comfort zone?

There is a popular saying that you mostly regret the things you did not do. And as I get older, I find this to be very true. Sure, I haven't always made the best choices in life, but who has? Hindsight is a wonderful thing, but as I look back on the choices I have made so far, there is no regret. There is a lot of learning and many great stories.

> *"A smooth sea never made a skilled sailor."*
>
> Franklin D Roosevelt

We will die without ever being sure we have reached our full potential. One way to explore your limits is to get out of your comfort zone and push yourself and see how far you can go. Try something new or do something that scares you a little.

There are so many amazing people in this world doing extraordinary things, and we look at them and say things like, "Wow, that's amazing, I could never do that". But is that true? Go back to Chapter 1 where I talk about limiting beliefs. There are people who are doing extraordinary things but they don't stop continuing to push themselves. One person who I admire is Courtney Dauwalter, an amazing ultrarunner who is also incredibly humble about her achievements. She keeps pushing herself to see what she is capable of, running days and days on end at astonishing speed. She keeps pushing the limits of what is possible, and she is an incredible inspiration.

As for my own experiences, I still can't believe that I have completed long distance triathlons and multi-day ultramarathons across tough terrain. I am not an athlete, far from it, but I am willing to stretch myself and see what I am capable of. If you had told me back in 2005 that I would do these things, I would have laughed. Now, I look back and I am proud of the things I have done, and I am excited about what the future can bring. There are no regrets, just lots of amazing memories.

Find your potential in what you consider to be near impossible.

"If you're always trying to be normal, you will never know how amazing you can be."
Maya Angelou

Be an inspiration

Do you have children or grandchildren? Do you want to inspire them and be a good role model? Children can develop and grow at an astonishing rate. From birth through to adolescence, they change physically, mentally and emotionally. As we reach adulthood, such development slows down. So, ask yourself, when was the last time you recognised a change in your emotional or mental growth? Have you completed studies, learned a new skill, climbed a mountain or discovered better ways to communicate with your significant other

97

to create a deeper, more meaningful relationship? Have you done something to make your children or grandchildren proud?

One of my favourite stories is about an American woman, Sabrina Pasterski, who, at the age of nine, had flown an aeroplane. She told a teacher of that accomplishment and the teacher responded with "That's nice, but what have you done lately?" Sabrina then went on to build a plane at the age of 12, continued to build her skills, received a doctorate in physics from Harvard at the age of 25 and is now regarded as a world-leading physicist. She uses the teacher's question of "What have you done lately?" as her mantra to continue to learn and grow. Sabrina's story is a reminder that we should all look for ways to be better than we were yesterday, to learn to grow and become better versions of ourselves.

Are you surviving or thriving?

Our time on this earth is limited and we don't know how long we have got. You really only have one brief shot at being the best that you can be on this planet yet we all have the ability to create whatever reality we desire. So why not be the most amazing person you can be?

Many of us, however, get so caught up in trying to please other people. We would rather try to please other people and do what is expected of us than do what we believe feels right and be the best we can be, whatever that looks like.

When I lived in the Middle East, sadly I went to quite a few funerals. People in their late 40s and early 50s, arguably in the prime of their life. They were cyclists, runners, triathletes. They were parents, brothers, sisters, sons, daughters. They were amazing human beings. They were living their best life and then it was cruelly cut short. I often think about those people and wonder what they would be doing now if they were still alive? We do not know when our time is up or if or when life will deal us a cruel blow.

I had my own serious health scare in 2012 when I was rushed to emergency with a pulmonary embolism, which is a life-threatening blood clot in the lung. I had experienced severe chest pain the night before I was due to run a half-marathon and I ended up at the local hospital, where I was misdiagnosed and sent home. I didn't do the half-marathon but I continued running a few other races in the following weeks, but I was incredibly breathless and couldn't understand why. It was only during a routine visit to my GP a few weeks later that he picked up that something serious was wrong with me and I was rushed to hospital and I am incredibly fortunate that I am still here today. It was a reminder that you never know when your time is up so take life by the horns, because you never know if or when you will get the chance again to do the things you want to do. And live with no regrets.

"Life begins at the end of your comfort zone."
Neale Donald Walsh

What does getting out of your comfort zone mean to you?

We all have different life experiences so what may be a stretch for one person may not be challenging to another.

One exercise you can do to assess what a stretch goal might look like to you is to find a quiet space with a pen and some paper (not your laptop or phone or other electronic device) and imagine that you are 95 years old and looking back on your life. What amazing things

STRETCH

have you accomplished? Brainstorm without any self-editing and write down whatever bubbles up in your thought process.

Another exercise is to think about the people you admire and whether you want to achieve the same things as them. It might be speaking a different language or two. It could be climbing Mt Kilimanjaro. Maybe you have always dreamed of walking the Camino de Santiago. Have you always thought of yourself as a funny person but have been too scared to try stand-up comedy? Think about the things that you would like to do but have always put off, for whatever reason.

> *"Two roads diverged in a wood, and I, I took the one less travelled by, and that has made all the difference."*
> Robert Frost

My story

Back in 2007, I was a recently divorced, childless woman in her thirties who wasn't loving the job she was doing in Sydney. Then I had an amazing opportunity in the form of a job in the Middle East. Despite considering myself as a reasonably well-educated adult, I was very ignorant about life in the Middle East and my opinion was shaded by news stories from that region which seemed to always be about conflict and death. I hesitated for some time about whether the job was worth it, as I was fearful about what life would be like living there. I travelled to Dubai in 2007 for the interview and was taken aback by how fast-paced, vibrant, multicultural, modern and extraordinary the place was. It was nothing like the news stories! And I took a leap of faith. I packed up my life in Sydney, sold my car, motorbike and Vespa and thought, well, I'll give it two years and see what happens. I ended up staying for ten years. It was one of the most amazing chapters of my life and I wouldn't change that decision if I had the chance again. I made incredible friends from around the world, learnt so much about other cultures and I came back to Australia a better person for the experience. But what would have happened if I had decided to stay in Sydney back in 2007? What would my life have been like? I'm sure it would have been nice and comfortable, but most likely a very beige and suburban existence. I took a leap of faith and moved my whole life to another country and another culture and I was enriched by the experience. I'm so glad I got out of my comfort zone and didn't let fear dominate my decision-making.

But what does that mean for you? I'm not necessarily saying that you should pack up your life and move elsewhere. However, I suggest that you reflect on the times where you perhaps let an unfounded fear dominate your decision making.

> *"Be comfortable being uncomfortable."*
> Marcus Smith, Peter McWilliams,
> Jillian Michaels and others

Ideas

Here are some ideas for getting out of your comfort zone:

(a) Try a new activity every year. I set myself a goal every year to try something new. Some of the things I have done are learning to surf, completing a diploma in culinary arts, wakeboarding, getting my motorbike licence, pole-dancing, learning Italian, and weightlifting. None of these things may interest you but be curious about the world around you and see what types of things may enrich your life. If you are an active outdoors type of person, consider a variation on some of the activities that you are doing now. For example, if you are a runner or cyclist, have you thought about trying a triathlon? Most triathlon clubs have a short distance enticer event so newbies can try out the sport and see if they like it. If you are more bookish or studious, maybe consider some short courses either online or in person. Once you learn something, no one can take that knowledge away from you.

(b) Look for short courses that require a registration and preferably some form of payment. Commit to it by registering straight away, block out the time in your calendar and set up a reminder a week and a day before. Once you pay, you are more likely to go through with it.

(c) Do something new with a friend. Try a RedBalloon experience or something similar and go with a bunch of friends. There are lots of adventures and activities to choose from, such as kayaking, hot air ballooning, abseiling, dancing, flight lessons and photography.

(d) Join a social club. There is practically a club for every sport and hobby nowadays, be it bushwalking, yoga, snorkelling, foreign films, photography, theatre games or cosplay. There is sure to be a group somewhere that would be of interest to you. It's also a great way to meet new people. I suggest finding a group that isn't too large. It's easy to get lost and disappear in the sea of people in a large group and therefore it is easy to not be accountable. Remember the DARE principles. You need to be accountable.

(e) How many times do you say 'no' to invitations, suggestions or ideas? Whenever you say no, you are potentially missing an opportunity to discover something new and to develop and grow. Try saying 'yes' to more things in your life and you may be pleasantly surprised by what you discover.

(f) If you believe that you don't have enough time or money to try anything new, read Chapters 3 – Delete and 9 – Invest.

"Life moves pretty fast. If you don't stop and look around once in a while, you could miss it."

Ferris Bueller

Applying the DARE Model

Here is an example of how to apply the DARE Model:

My SMARTer lifestyle goal is…	It is 5 July 2022 and I am recognised as an accomplished public speaker.
The SMARTer habit goal that supports my lifestyle goal is…	I will attend the fortnightly Toastmasters sessions in my local area.
My **Desire** for achieving this habit goal is…	9/10
I will be **Accountable** by…	Paying my membership and committing to other members that I will turn up. Recording one five-minute video on the first day of each month and posting it to my YouTube channel and to Facebook. Posting a 15-second video on TikTok every Sunday morning.

I will **Reward** myself for doing this habit by…	For each TikTok video I post, I will go out for coffee or breakfast at a café afterwards.
The changes I will make to my **Environment** are…	Set up a tripod in my office so I can easily record videos on my mobile phone. Put post-it notes on my bathroom mirror as a prompt to practice speaking to the mirror when I do my makeup in the mornings.

CHAPTER 7

Connect

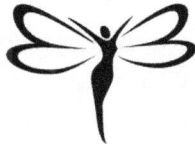

"Deep human connection is...the purpose and the result of a meaningful life – and it will inspire the most amazing acts of love, generosity and humanity."
Melinda Gates

Introduction

Ironically, as we become a more and more connected world, people have never felt lonelier. Recent surveys suggest that people are feeling more disconnected from family and friends. Even though we can reach out to anyone at any time through social media – platforms designed to connect people – we are feeling increasingly isolated. COVID-19 exacerbated this for many people, with forced lockdowns and restrictions on movement and on gatherings, separating families and friends. My uncle passed away in March 2020 and it was incredibly sad that only three people in my family could attend due to the restrictions on travel and gatherings. At a time when my family needed comfort and support, we were unable to be there for each other in person. To me, that really highlighted the importance of human connection, not just in grief, but in our everyday lives.

Why is social connection important?

Why do we need social connection? Humans are social creatures and have always relied on each other for our survival. Social connection is also critical for mental health. Having a sense of belonging and maintaining friendships with others provides a support network for us. Studies indicate that a lack of social support is on par with smoking cigarettes as a risk factor for morbidity and mortality and is considered even more harmful than other stressors, such as obesity and air pollution.[26]

Various studies have also shown that one of the keys to living a long and fulfilled life is to nurture strong social networks. For example, the people in Okinawa in Japan are known for living long lives. Okinawa is considered a Blue Zone. Blue Zones are areas of the world where a high proportion of people live much longer than average. In Okinawa, this is partly attributed to a tradition called Moai, which are support groups that are created in childhood and last for life. These secure social networks are considered as social 'safety nets', where members of the network provide emotional, spiritual and other support to each other in times of need. It provides a level of mental comfort knowing that there is always a support network there for you in good times and in bad, no matter what.

COVID-19 showed us that social connection is critical for wellbeing and that it is more meaningful when it is in person, not via social media. Despite being connected online with people, being physically isolated and distanced from others saw an increase in mental health concerns. Recent studies tend to confirm the view that social connection in the real (rather than virtual) world is vital for our wellbeing.[27] Other research has shown that extensive use of social media can build shallow, weak ties with others, increases self-focus such as narcissism, and may lead to mental health issues for some individuals. The same research goes on to indicate increased use of social media over time can cause a decline in empathy for others, in civic engagement, and in political involvement.[23]

Some of the benefits of real-world social connection include:

- Lower levels of anxiety, stress and depression
- Lower levels of cortisol
- Stronger immune system
- Better resilience
- Improved memory and focus
- Improved sleep
- Higher self-esteem
- More empathy with others

Interacting with others also provides a level of accountability when trying to form and adhere to positive habits. On top of that, it is a wonderful way to learn from others with different experiences which in turn enriches your own life (see Chapter 6 – Stretch on my Middle East experience).

What does your social network look like?

You may have heard the saying that you are the average of the five people you spend the most time with. It makes sense that the ideas and actions of the people you spend a lot of time with will rub off on you. But reflect on whether the people in your social circle have the same outlook on life as you do. If we go back to the DARE Model in Chapter 1, consider how your behaviours are influenced by the people you associate with. Do you drink too much alcohol on a Friday night because that's what your friends or colleagues do? Or do you get up early on a Saturday morning to go for a run because that is what that group of friends does?

A good friend should help make life more meaningful for you. But there may be people in your world who suck all the oxygen and energy out of your life. Think about your friendships and ask yourself:

- Do your friends continually criticise you or do they support you in what you do?
- Do they talk relentlessly about themselves in conversations but never offer a comforting shoulder in return?
- Do they discredit and undermine you or do they offer constructive feedback instead?
- Do they always find a way to make the conversation about them or are they empathetic and supportive when you are going through difficult times?

Many of us have toxic people in our friendship circle, people who can and will bring us down instead of providing us with emotional and moral support. The consequence of having such people in your life is that it can increase your stress levels, you can feel incredibly alone, and it can also adversely affect the positive friendships that you do have.

So what should you do?

A friendship with a toxic person is a tricky thing to navigate. You may want to try to repair the friendship by talking openly with the other person about your concerns. Alternatively, you can consider ending the friendship or reducing your interactions with them. There is no right or wrong answer. Ultimately, you will have to weigh up whether that person is an important part of your life or not. If their role in your life is affecting your mental health, then consider seeking professional support and help.

Another thing to consider is that if you are seeking fulfilling and meaningful connections, this is generally more sustainable with a handful of people in your life than it is with a large group.

My story

I like to think of my friendship circle as quality over quantity. I have many acquaintances, but a small but tightknit circle of friends. My friends are people who share similar values to me, and I know that if one of us was in distress, we could pick up the phone and call each other at 3.00 am and be there for each other, fully and completely.

While we can be connected to people via social media or on Zoom calls – particularly during COVID-19 lockdowns and restrictions – this should be considered as an additional way to connect with others, not the only way. Research has shown the importance of real-life human connection as having many benefits, particularly for our mental health. When I was in the middle of the desert doing multi-day ultramarathons, the race organisers made it clear that use of mobile devices was forbidden, unless you needed to use it for an emergency. The consequence of this is that at the end of each day, runners gathered in camp and met other people with similar interests but with diverse backgrounds and experiences and we chatted around campfires instead of burying our heads in our mobile phones. We learnt about each other and our families and we had serious, meaningful and philosophical conversations as well as lots of laughs. It was certainly one of the highlights of these events for me. I met many amazing people and I am still in contact with many of them.

A German tale

There is an extraordinary story about unexpected friendships that can form in local communities. The story is from Kotti, a suburb of Berlin. The area was a mix of marginalised groups – Muslim immigrants, gay activists, and punk squatters. After the fall of the Berlin Wall, house prices skyrocketed and as a result many tenants who lived in social housing in Kotti saw their rents increase significantly. Many people could not afford to pay and a number of them were evicted. One such person was an elderly disabled Muslim woman, Nuriye Cengiz, who had pinned a sign in her window facing the street that said, "I got my eviction notice, so I will be thrown out next week. Therefore on Thursday, I am going to kill myself."

Many of the residents came to see Nuriye to offer support and help but she refused. What followed was an extraordinary tale of unexpected friendships. The residents demanded a rent freeze for the whole estate and demanded that Nuriye could stay in her flat. Neighbours came together and blocked the main road through Kotti and they barricaded the area outside Nuriye's flat for months and worked together as a community, united in their desire to help Nuriye. This attracted significant media attention. Over that time, an unlikely friendship formed between the elderly Muslim woman Nuriye and a punk squatter named Tanya. As mentioned, the community of Kotti was diverse – punk women in miniskirts and very religious Muslim women, old white males and gay colourful men, Muslim men and gay women.[24] Tanya and others in the neighbourhood guarded the barricades in rotating shifts to ensure the police would not tear down the barricades when there was no one there to keep watch. When Tanya was on watch, the conversations with Nuriye were awkward as they struggled to find anything in common. But one night they discovered they had a similar story. Both women had children at a young age and were living in difficult circumstances after migrating from Turkey to Germany. They both realised that they had been children with children of their own, struggling to make ends meet in a foreign country. A bond had been formed and a friendship between the unlikely pair developed. And the story has a happy ending – Nuriye got to stay in her apartment.

Ideas

As mentioned, your behaviours are influenced by the people you associate with. If you are trying to form positive habits, then that can mean reassessing who you spend time with. As a result, that can mean that people will exit our lives and new people will come into our lives. However, for many people, making new friends requires special effort, especially as an adult. Maintaining healthy friendships also takes some diligence and care. But remember that true friendships can be one of the most rewarding aspects of our lives.

Here are some ideas:

(a) Seek out opportunities to connect with people, even in a small way. For example, if you are in the supermarket, consider joining the queue at the checkout with people waiting to be served, rather than using the self-checkout, and speak to the people in front of you or behind you. Engage in a chat with the checkout operator. Ask their name or refer to their name if they are wearing a name badge. That may sound minor and a bit odd, but humans generally experience an increase in their mood after having a positive interaction with another person and it can help us feel more connected to our local community.

(b) While it can sometimes be daunting to meet new people, showing curiosity and interest in other people will often open up something in common and pave the way for interesting conversations. Take the pressure off yourself, focus on the other person and be a keen listener. I for one am always looking for ways to be a better listener as this is a key factor in making deeper connections with other people. One of the greatest gifts you can give someone else is to turn up, listen, and be present. Don't look at your phone every few minutes when you are talking with someone and place your attention on the other person and on what they are saying. Don't formulate a response in your head while the other person is talking and instead ask follow-up questions to get a better understanding of them and their story. Your goal should be to listen with the intention of understanding the other person, and this is the essence of active listening. There are many great resources out there on active listening and I encourage you to continue to improve this skill. It can really deepen your connection with other people.

(c) Get out of your comfort zone and be willing to try something new, such as joining a club, signing up for a course, or pursuing activities that you're interested in, as this provides the opportunity to meet like-minded people. Start small, such as by going to a different gym class to the one that you usually attend or even initiating a simple conversation with a stranger at a café. Say yes to things more often, even if you initially are not that interested.

(d) How about your neighbours? How well do you know them? I live in a complex with eight families and we all know each other, we know each other's names and the names of our pets, and we all get along. We also help each other out in times of need, such as by looking after each other's pets if we are away for a few days. It's a lovely, harmonious environment and yet we are all from different backgrounds with the ages of the adults ranging from 20 to 70+ years. What is the secret? I think the answer is fairly simple. We are interested in each other as people and we care about our small community. It's the glue that binds. Do you know your neighbours? Would they be able to help out if you were in need? And would you know if they needed your help?

(e) Another way to develop your sense of connection to others is to volunteer your time and to do something for someone else. This has been shown to lead to increased happiness. This could be as simple as getting a coffee for a colleague without them asking. Or it could be donating blood or plasma. One of the great things that the Red Cross blood donor centres in Australia (and elsewhere in the world) do is when your donation is used, you receive a text message saying that your blood product has been used at a particular hospital for a patient in need. This can help people feel a connection with the world around us.

(f) If you are looking for inspiration, check out the heart-warming documentary called Old People's Home for 4 Year Olds, a documentary that brings elderly people into a classroom of pre-schoolers. The experiment endeavours to see if this simple interaction can improve the lives of the participants, particularly as social isolation and loss of connection with their community are some of the biggest challenges for the elderly.

Applying the DARE Model

So how can we apply the DARE Model? Here is an example that may help you generate your own ideas.

My SMARTer lifestyle goal is…	It is 30 June 2022 and I have improved my sense of belonging in my new community by at least 50%.
The SMARTer habit goal that supports my lifestyle goal is…	I will join my local book club and attend every month.
My **Desire** for achieving this habit goal is…	7/10.
I will be **Accountable** by…	Joining the book club and committing to other members that I will go. Posting my attendance on social media.
I will **Reward** myself for doing this habit by…	Buying myself a new lipstick after I attend my first book club and buying myself a new perfume when I attend four meetings in a row.
The changes I will make to my **Environment** are…	Block out at least 30 minutes a day in my calendar to read the monthly book of choice. Place the book in obvious places e.g. bedside, handbag, and download onto my tablet.

CHAPTER 8

Move

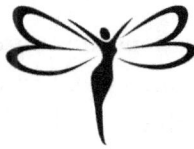

"Exercise is a celebration of what your body can do, not a punishment for what you ate."

Unknown

Introduction

Why do we exercise? That may sound like a strange question, but we all have different reasons for exercising.[25] It could be because we want to be fit and healthy. Maybe we want to change our body composition, reduce our body fat and add lean muscle. It may be to support our mental health, and many studies show the importance of physical activity in supporting positive mental health. It could be to reduce the risk as we age of developing metabolic disease such as type 2 diabetes and obesity or for mature women in particular, to help with maintaining bone density. Or it could be vanity. For me, I love the fact that I have toned and defined back, shoulder and arm muscles and that boosts my self-confidence. I've worked hard for those muscles. I didn't borrow, steal, or buy them. I earned them, and it makes me feel great.

My story

I love to exercise and to move. I especially love to be in nature, so any chance I get to go for a bushwalk or a swim in the ocean, I am there!

Over the years I have done various running events, including a number of ultramarathons as mentioned in Chapter 3 across the Sahara and Gobi Deserts. They are tough events, but I loved completing them as not only did I meet the most amazing human beings but I also realised that I was able to achieve something that I never thought was possible.

I have different reasons for exercising:

(a) I want to still have good mobility and strength as I get older.
(b) I want to see what I am capable of achieving.
(c) I enjoy seeing the positive changes to my body.
(d) I enjoy exercising!

What's your why?

> *"Rather than focusing on the results of a habit, focus on how it makes you feel…Exercising to look better isn't sustainable, the daily effect is too small. Exercise to feel better. It works every day."*
>
> James Clear

Do you want to lose weight?

In Chapter 5 – Nourish I talked about the importance of a healthy diet and how you can make better dietary choices.

If your reason for exercising is to lose weight then I have a newsflash for you. You can't outtrain a bad diet. Exercise alone will not help you lose weight. You really need to get your food intake right first. You could exercise for three hours a day and burn 1,200 calories, then consume 3,500 calories, and you will still be in a calorie surplus, not a deficit. If you ate a burger and some fries and a soft drink for lunch, that would probably be around 4,000 calories and you would need to run a half marathon, or 21 kilometres, to burn off those calories. But even if you burned off those calories through exercise, you are not reversing the negative effects that poor food choices can have on your body such as your gut microbiome. So it's not just about the calories you eat, but it is also about the other negative impacts on your health that you can't exercise away.

Simply put, if you consume more calories than you burn you won't lose weight.

Spot reducing

One of the biggest myths is that you need to do abdominal exercises to lose body fat in your belly area. The fact is you can't spot reduce body fat. You can certainly tone particular areas of your body by increasing muscle in that area, but that does not equate to reducing body fat in that area.

This means that while exercise will certainly help to find your abdominal muscles, if you want to see what they look like under that layer of belly fat, you need to actually manage your calories through dietary intake. Nutrient-dense foods that are closest to their natural form are best, because they will help you feel fuller for longer, and will also provide you with nutrition that you need and help maintain or reduce any cravings you may have for less nutritious foods. Many fast foods contain sugars and hydrogenated fat, giving you empty calories as you obtain little to no nutritional benefit.

Understanding how your body uses energy

How much energy do you burn each day and how much of that relates to structured exercise activity? The answer may surprise you.

There are four main ways that our body burns energy (or calories). They are:

(a) BMR – this stands for basal metabolic rate
(b) NEAT – this stands for non-exercise activity thermogenesis
(c) TEF – this stands for the thermic effect of food
(d) EAT – this stands for your exercise activity thermogenesis.

BMR is the number of calories that your body burns at rest. So even while you are lying down, you are burning calories to keep you alive. It's the energy that goes into your heart pumping blood around the body, for your lungs to take in and expel air and the energy it takes to grow hair and regenerate skin cells. Your BMR consists of about 60-70% of the calories you burn each day.

NEAT is the number of calories that you burn from incidental movement, such as moving around the house or office, hanging out the washing, standing while you are working at a sit and stand desk, or walking up some stairs. It is non-structured exercise and makes up about 15% of the calories you burn each day.

TEF is the thermic effect of food. This refers to the calories your body burns in order to digest the food you eat, which involves things such as breaking it down, digesting it and absorbing it into the bloodstream. It makes up about 10% of the energy you burn each day.

EAT is the energy you burn from structured activity, such as running, swimming, doing a HIIT class or lifting weights. It makes up about 10-15% of the energy you burn each day.

Obviously, these percentages will vary from one person to the next and will be influenced by various factors, such as your age, state of health and level of activity (for example, nurses and teachers and other professionals and workers who perform jobs that have a physical aspect will have a higher percentage of calories burned from NEAT or EAT).

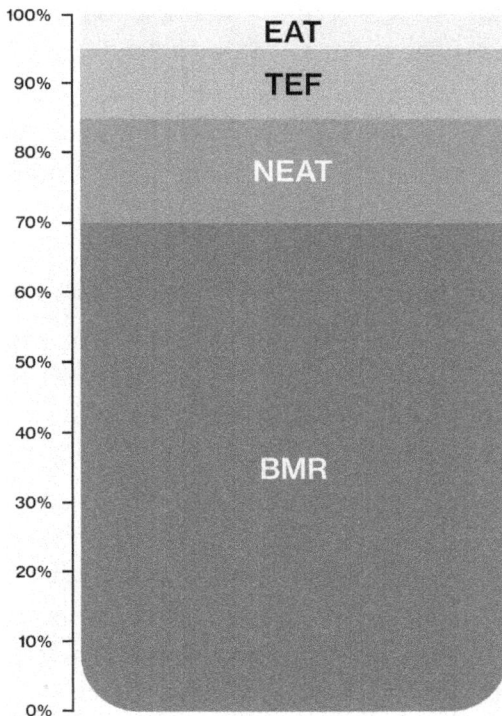

So EAT activities such as going to the gym or going for a run or bike ride are great and will help you get fitter and healthier, but the amount of energy you burn from exercise is relatively low compared to your BMR. If weight loss is your goal, look closely at your diet and understand how many calories you consume each day, as that is where you will really see the most impact on your overall weight loss. Continue to exercise, and in particular consider adding more NEAT to your day, such as incidental walking. Strength training can also help raise your BMR, as you will develop lean muscle mass, and the more lean muscle you have, the higher your BMR.

How much should I exercise?

How much you should exercise depends on your goals. If you want to run a marathon, you will need to condition your body to be able to run 42.2 kilometres and you can only do that by putting in the time and effort, which can mean ten or more hours a week. The level and intensity of activity will also depend on whether your goal is simply to finish or to complete the marathon in a competitive time.

If you want to complete a full distance triathlon – a 3.8 km swim, followed by a 180 km cycle then a marathon, all in under 16 hours – you will need to train across three sports for several months, with training hours of 15-20 hours or more a week. When I trained for my first full distance triathlon, I was training 25 hours a week in my peak training phase. So it really does depend on what your goals are.

Unless you are training for a particularly demanding event such as a full distance triathlon, then more is not necessarily better. Consistency is usually more important than volume. You don't need to be vigorously working out five hours a day, seven days a week. For most people, moderate activity for 30 minutes a day, several times a week, is all you need to be doing.

It is in our nature to keep moving, not to be sitting in front of a television or mobile device for hours on end watching mindless content. We are designed to move and I heard this fantastic saying recently that 'motion is lotion'. In other words, we need to keep moving to keep our joints and muscles happy.

There's also a belief that you must exercise for at least an hour for it to be of benefit. Unfortunately, this allows for all the excuses to start. Let me paint a picture. It's 6.00 pm and you've just got home from work. Your mind is buzzing with all the things that you think you need to do. Pay bills. Make dinner. Wash up. Iron some clothes. All these chores that stand between you and the gym. So you think, "I can't afford the one and a half hours it will take for me to get ready, go to the gym, workout, come home, and shower, so I just won't go". But who loses in all of this? You do. You miss out on doing something active. Another way of looking at this could be, "It's 6.00 pm and I have chores to do but I will find 20 minutes to exercise. I will put my tray bake dinner in the oven and while that is cooking, I will go for a 20-minute walk or run."

It is usually better to do less than you planned than to do absolutely nothing at all. Another approach is to break exercise down into smaller chunks, especially if you have not exercised in a while. 15 minutes of walking a day, every day, is better than doing nothing. Try adding a short walk after lunch. Benefits of this include improved mental focus, better mood, more energy, improved fat loss and better digestion.

People who say they have no time for exercise usually don't have a strong enough desire to be active. If you really do care about your health and fitness, then you will make time in your day for it. If you exercise for 30 minutes a day, that is only 2% of your day. Yes, you read that right. 2%. How can you create space in your day to exercise? See also Chapter 3 – Delete.

"I trained for four years to run nine seconds. Some people don't see results in two months and give up."

Usain Bolt

What exercise should I do?

Many people whose aim is to get fit think that they need to run. But what if you don't like running? Well, if you don't enjoy running then don't do it. Find an exercise that you enjoy doing. You are then more likely to view exercise as a pleasurable activity and stick with it over time. I used to enjoy running and then I had a number of injuries and developed a chronic condition called a Morton's neuroma, so I had to take a break from any impact sports, such as running. So I took a break from running and I shifted my mindset from "what can't I do" to "what can I do". I then took up weightlifting, which I am really enjoying. And funnily enough, during the process of writing this book, I managed to break my big toe by dropping a weight plate on my foot. It meant that I wasn't able to go to the gym for several weeks. I then spoke to my trainer about adjusting my program, so I could come back and at least do upper body work, because I missed the gym so much. It had become a regular habit, something that was ingrained in me, and not being able to go was frustrating. It was a reminder again that language and mindset are important and that exercise is not punishment for what you ate. Exercise is a blessing. The language I used wasn't "I have to work out" but "I get to work out". A simple shift in language and in mindset moves exercise from being a burden to exercise being a positive experience. Look at a habit as a way to build skills, rather than a challenge, as this will make the habit more attractive.

122

Children tend to be quite active, playing sports at school and outside school, engaging in physical games like hide and seek, and just playing such as having fun on the monkey bars at the local park. As we get older, our level of activity tends to reduce. Life gets busy, we get a mortgage, we work hard, and we often neglect the opportunity to be physically active. If we have children, sometimes we don't have those activity-based interactions with them. Exercising with your kids not only has physical benefits but it also gives you an opportunity to engage more fully with them and can help families thrive.

The importance of rest

While exercise is important to develop fitness and gain lean muscle, that is not how we get stronger. We get stronger through recovery. Rest and sleep are important components in being healthy and stronger. You need balance in all aspects of your life. This also includes mental health and human connection. See Chapter 11 – Restore and Chapter 7 – Connect.

Ideas

Here are some ideas on how to kickstart your exercise journey:

1. Start small and keep going (see my story in Chapter 1 about my running journey after my divorce).

2. Build exercise into your day with incidental activity, for example, park your car further away from the shopping centre entrance or get off the bus a stop earlier and walk the rest of the distance to your destination.

3. Connect with someone with similar goals for support and accountability (see also Chapter 7 – Connect).

4. Put out your gym clothing and prepare your gym bag and water bottle the night before if you plan to exercise the following morning.

5. Place a calendar in a visible place with ticks/crosses when workout or exercise is done/not done.

6. After lunch, go for a 10-minute walk. This is also an example of piggybacking off an existing practice – eating a meal.

7. Block out time in your calendar for exercise and stick to it. Treat it as you would a business meeting or family commitment – do not cancel!

8. If you don't have a pet, then offer to take a neighbour's dog for a walk.

9. If you live or work in a building with lifts, then use the stairs instead for at least a few flights. I used to live on the 33rd floor of a building and I would sometimes get out of the lift on a lower floor then walk the rest of the way.

Applying the DARE Model

Here is an example of how we could apply the DARE Model to move more:

My SMARTer lifestyle goal is…	It is 3 March 2022 and I am exercising at least 30 minutes a day, 5 times a week.
The SMARTer habit goal that supports my lifestyle goal is…	I will do the HIIT class at my local gym every Tuesday and Friday morning.
My **Desire** for achieving this habit goal is…	8/10.
I will be **Accountable** by…	Telling my best friend and gym buddy and encouraging her to join me. Posting my workouts on social media.
I will **Reward** myself for doing this habit by…	Buying some new leggings or top for every month I consistently hit my habit goal between now and 3 March 2022.
The changes I will make to my **Environment** are…	Put out my gym clothes the night before so I can get ready easily in the morning before class.

Before embarking on any new exercise regime, consult with your doctor or health care professional.

CHAPTER 9

Invest

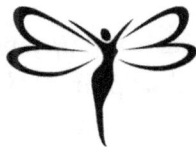

"Someone is sitting in the shade today because someone planted a tree a long time ago."

Warren Buffet

Introduction

Research from the National Australia Bank (**NAB**) showed that 40% of Australians were experiencing some form of financial stress or hardship in late 2019, the highest number of financially stressed Australians since Q4 2016, and an increase from 36% in Q3 2019.[26] Many people in Australia were already battling drought and catastrophic bushfires and then in 2020 the COVID-19 pandemic saw the number of people experiencing financial distress climb even further. Many people did not have a safety net of cash to help them ride through tough times, and in 2020, a record $36 billion of superannuation savings was withdrawn by nearly 3 million Australians, which will have its own long-term financial impacts on those individuals.

In the NAB survey, the main reason for financial distress was cited as not having enough money for an emergency, followed by being unable to pay bills (19%), not having enough money for food and essentials (16%) and an inability to pay for medical bills (11%). Sadly, the number of women experiencing hardship jumped to 42%, up from 35% in Q3 2019, but remained relatively stable for men at 38% (slightly up from 37% in Q3 2019).

What would you do if a sudden and unexpected life event meant that your main source of income disappeared? Would you be in a position to continue paying your bills and meeting your other financial obligations? If so, for how long? Was COVID-19 a wakeup call for you?

Many people would not be able to survive more than a few weeks without their main source of income. So how do you protect yourself from the negative impact of an event that is beyond your control? What impact will it have on your life and how do you establish a financially secure future?

The gender gap

Not having enough money to ride out an emergency is particularly an issue for women, who may have had career breaks or are more likely to work part-time, and generally earn less than men. This is compounded by the fact that lower income then means a smaller amount is contributed to superannuation, given that an employer's contribution to superannuation is set at a percentage of the employee's income, so the more you earn, the more money will go into superannuation from your employer. An article in the Sydney Morning Herald explains that "The gender pay gap is the difference between women and men's average full-time weekly salaries, expressed as a percentage of men's salaries. The gender pay gap has remained relatively stable in Australia for close to two decades, with 2018 being the first year it dropped below 15 per cent...The gender pay gap in Australia (as of August 2018) is 14.6 per cent, which equates to a woman earning, on average, $244.80 less than men each week."[27]

As a result, women have substantially lower superannuation savings than men. A 2020 Canstar report shows that the superannuation balance of Australian women in their 40s and 50s are $107,000-$180,000 short of what is needed for a comfortable retirement.[28] Inequity in superannuation balances largely arise from inequities during working life.

Furthermore, women over 55 are the fastest growing group of homeless people in Australia. There are more than 300,000 women between 45 and 65 years of age who are at significant risk of homelessness when they retire, and two thirds of single retired Australian women over 65 currently live below the poverty line.[29] These are grim statistics.

The impact of not having enough savings can lead to financial struggles in retirement or even not being able to retire until you are in your seventies or eighties as you can't afford to stop working. This is not the same as choosing to continue to work because you enjoy what you do. The issue is where you must continue to work to pay bills and survive. Do you really want to be working in your seventies and eighties if you don't want to? And do you want to live a life where there is constant worry and stress about money and your financial security?

Superannuation

In Australia, superannuation is a way of saving for retirement and consists of money put aside by a person's employer (together with any contributions made by the employee) into an investment fund over a person's working life. It is essentially a form of forced savings. The amount can't generally be accessed until you reach retirement age. Currently, Australian law mandates an amount that an employer must contribute to super, which at the time of writing is 9.5% of an employee's salary. An employee can also make contributions, the most common way being to divert pre-tax salary, which is a tax-effective way for saving, especially for those on high income tax thresholds, as superannuation is taxed at 15%, while the highest income tax bracket at the time of writing is 49%. Your superannuation fund then invests the money in a range of assets (such as Australian or international shares, property, bonds and term deposits). Depending on your year of birth, you can access your superannuation after 55 years of age. Superannuation is complex and is governed by a range of regulatory rules so before making any changes to your superannuation, consult a financial advisor or accountant who can provide you with tailored financial advice specific to your circumstances and to your risk profile. The Australian Tax Office's website also has an abundance of information about Australian superannuation.

My suggestion to you though is to consider what additional contributions you can make to your superannuation as this will impact the amount of money with which you can retire. It builds your potential for investment growth and also utilises the power of compound interest over time and the older you get, the harder it will be to catch up.

Compound interest is essentially the process of earning interest on interest. So money invested in super would earn interest on the money that is contributed, plus you also earn interest on the interest you earned. Over the passage of time, this is a powerful way to build wealth. So a 25-year-old putting an extra $50 a month into super will have an extra $175,000 by age 65, while a 35-year-old who did the same would have an extra $79,000 and a 45-year-old would have $32,000. Master the art of delayed gratification in order to see a return on any of your investments.

If you are an employee, discuss with your financial advisor the most effective way to top up your superannuation. If you are self-employed, then also seek out the services of a professional advisor and consider contributing 10% of your earnings into a superannuation scheme.

"The more your money works for you, the less you have to work for money."

Idowu Koyenikan

Invest in yourself

My mantra has always been to invest in yourself first, a variation on Robert Kiyosaki's saying of pay yourself first.[30] What does that mean though? For me, this means putting money aside for my future before I spend it on anything else. It means investing it in different places to diversify the risk so I can build my wealth without requiring any extra effort from me.

Understand the difference between earning money and making money. Earning money is when you perform a job and you are paid a wage or salary. Making money is what you do with those earnings, such as investing it.

I have a practice of transferring funds out of my main bank account into an investment account that is held with another financial institution. Why do I do that? Well, that secondary account is never touched. I don't use it for any payments or transactions. It is merely there to collect my savings and the funds are directed to a variety of investments such as international and domestic shares and property trusts. My risk profile has been assessed as being 'moderate growth' which is relatively risk-averse, so my investments are based on that risk profile. If I were younger, perhaps my risk profile, and therefore my investment strategy, may be more aggressive, but at this stage of my life I am looking for solid growth, not significant (and slightly riskier) gains. Over time, my investment has steadily grown and because I don't see it regularly or have direct access to it, I am often surprised when I do check on my balance and see it is growing nicely without me having to work harder or longer.

I also have a savings account that I call my 'play money' or rainy day money. While the investment account is for continued financial growth to help me as I approach semi-retirement and retirement, the savings account is where I transfer a (smaller) set amount each month, again into another bank account with another bank, which makes it harder for me to access and easier to set and forget. The funds in the savings account are there as a safety net in case an emergency arises, for example, if I suddenly became ill and was unable to work, or to pay for luxuries such as a deluxe holiday or a home renovation. Over time, I have steadily accumulated a tidy amount of money in my savings and every 12-18 months, I assess and decide what I may do with it. If I don't use it as 'play money', I will consider moving it to another form of investment, such as shares. With banks offering very low interest rates in 2021, I am now looking at other places to park my savings, as a bank account is not going to provide me with much of a return, but I still ensure that I put money aside each month for that rainy or sunny day.

That then means that my main bank account is used to pay my bills and expenses with whatever money I have left after I have put my investment and savings aside. I have to make do with whatever is left, but I always, always pay myself first.

But I hear you say that you have debts, a mortgage etc., so how can you possibly save? Even if it is a small amount, get into the habit of paying yourself first on a regular basis. It is the consistency over time that will make a difference. And if you have children, get them into this habit because the earlier you start, the better, as you can then utilise the power of compound interest, although in 2021, this is not likely to be much – if anything! But the philosophy here is to be patient and to build up a financial asset over time. Many people also view saving money as a sacrifice or a challenge, but if you flip your mindset to instead view savings as a way to create a financially secure future, then that can set you up for success.

What I find works for me is to automate as much as possible. I have set up automatic monthly transfers from my main bank account to my savings account and to my investment fund and I don't even notice it is gone. I have then found a way to manage on whatever is left.

I don't have money to invest!

I often hear people say that investing is only for rich people, or you need a lot of money to invest, but that is not true. The simplest way to build wealth is to invest, no matter how small an investment you make. One simple example is buying shares. In Australia, the minimum order size for shares for your first order is generally quite small, such as a minimum of $500 worth of shares. Investing in shares gives you two ways to make money – by capital growth as the share price grows over time, and by dividends, which are payments of a portion of a company's profits that are made to its shareholders. If you look at the performance of some of the blue-chip companies in Australia over the past five years – such as Fortescue Metals, Woolworths and Macquarie Group – you will see that their share prices have steadily climbed. If you had bought shares in these companies five years ago, you would have doubled your investment. Unfortunately, past performance is not an indicator of future performance, so always do your homework first and if you are unsure, seek out the advice of a professional. Also be aware that if you sell shares at a profit, you may be liable to capital gains tax. Again, seek out the advice of a financial professional.

There is also a difference between investing in shares and trading in shares. An investment is usually held for a longer period with an expectation of growth over time. Trading is more speculative and traders typically only hold shares for short periods of time, such as a day or less. While there is nothing wrong with trading as such, it does come with higher risks and you really need to know what you are doing.

If you don't believe shares are a good option for you, then consider other ways to build your finances, such as a side gig. Creating some form of passive income such as from your own online course in the area of your expertise can create some passive income for you.

If buying your own home and having a mortgage is currently outside of your reach, you could consider being what's called a rentvestor. This is where you would buy a home in an area that is more affordable and rent it out, while renting in the area where you currently work and live. At the time of writing, rents in Australian capital cities, especially in Sydney, have come down. So that may be a strategy that you could consider. Don't forget to invest in yourself as well, whether that means further education or learning additional skills to add to your toolkit, as this can increase your earning potential.

If you have some savings, that's great, but this isn't particularly helpful if interest rates are low, as they currently are in 2021, so they will not offer the best return on your investment. Simply saving your money is not enough. At the time of writing, the interest rate on a five-year term deposit of between $5,000 and $49,999 was just 0.25%. Find ways to make your money work harder for you, even while you are asleep, whether it is investing in shares or some other form of investment that will help grow your money over the long-term. You need to take a long-term view – even if your assets are growing at say 3% a year – as it can make a material difference over a longer period of time due to the power of compounding.

Another thing I hear, particularly from people in their forties and fifties, is that it is too late. Yes, the earlier you start to invest, the longer you have to allow your investments to grow over time. But why not start now? If you put aside $50 a week, you will have $2,600 after a year, putting you in a better financial position than you are now. And if you don't put aside that money? Well a year from now you will be another year older but without those savings, so what are you waiting for? If you are able to invest it wisely, it could be worth even more. Over time, this will continue to build and grow. Just get started, and get started now, as this will allow time for your investment to work harder for you.

But I don't know how to invest!

I must admit that in my younger days, I wasn't that savvy when it came to investments. Yes, I have a Commerce degree, but that doesn't necessarily translate into knowing the practical day-to-day aspects of how to build your financial future. But I was (and still am) a keen learner. I attended courses on how to invest in shares. I bought books like Rich Dad Poor Dad[31], The Barefoot Investor[32] and Trend

Trading[33] to learn more about practical ways to help build wealth. And also my ex-husband and I shared the same outlook – we wanted the option of an early retirement! We were keen property investors and when we divorced, we divided up our property investments and I still hold some of those properties today. My motivation over the years hasn't really changed. I am still keen on an early retirement or a semi-retirement and I want the option to stop working if and when I choose to. Fortunately for me, I am now in that situation. I can choose to step back from the rat race, knowing that I have enough assets behind me to sustain me for the years ahead. But I continue to work because I love what I do. I have a choice that not many other people have, thanks largely to having built great financial habits from a young age.

My advice is to be curious and to learn about money and investments, particularly if you are a woman. I have met many women over the years who have relied on their partner to look after the money side of their relationship. I have also met women who, after a divorce or the premature death of their spouse, are clueless about their financial situation. They struggle to make ends meet, and I have even met people who have no idea how to manage a mortgage or pay bills. Be in control of your financial destiny. Having financial agency is one of the most powerful things you can do. And if you have a significant other, then discuss your financial goals and strategies together. Be engaged in the process and be willing to learn.

If you're looking for ideas on how to invest, then do your homework. There are lots of wonderful resources and informative websites that you can learn from. But be discerning in which ones you choose to read. Follow a mix of different people who are regarded as experts in the financial arena to get an idea of what investment options may be suitable for you.

Before you start, you must also have a clear investment strategy. Let's go back to our SMART goals in Chapter 2 – Evaluate. To be effective, goals need to be specific, measurable, achievable, relevant and time-based. Without a plan, you are likely to fail.

What about a financial advisor?

In my early forties I engaged the services of a financial advisor and it was one of the best things I have done. Unfortunately, there are some in the industry who are unscrupulous, but I have been fortunate in that I trust mine implicitly with my investments and I trust the advice he gives me. But I also read everything he sends me, I sometimes question and challenge the advice he gives me and I make sure I understand what his recommendations involve before I proceed with any changes to my investments. I also make sure I understand what fees I pay and how they are calculated. I do not outsource the decision-making responsibility to him. I am still informed and remain responsible for my financial decisions. What I have found is that a financial advisor can help you with understanding your risk profile and what your appetite for risk is. I have also been active in learning more about finances so I can make informed decisions about my financial future.

Spending

It's fantastic if you are able to squirrel away money into investments, but what about the spending side of the equation?

Housing has generally been considered to be the largest household expense in Australia, followed by household bills and expenses such as utility bills, insurance and groceries. It is estimated that the average

Australian household spends about $300 a week on food and groceries, which is a significant expense.

One thing that I stay on top of is my spending patterns. I identify where I am perhaps spending more than I should and I then redistribute or re-prioritise my spending as necessary. I use my credit card for just about every purchase. This works for me but may not work for everyone. The first reason I do this is so I don't have to think about carrying cash with me. Secondly, my credit card has a great rewards program and I use the points I accumulate in the rewards program to pay for various things. I buy all of my petrol vouchers through the rewards program and I recently bought a Dyson vacuum cleaner and some lovely designer earrings through the same rewards program. Thirdly, my bank has a feature on their online banking that will give me a breakdown of the different categories of spending such as groceries, bills and utilities, dining out and fuel. Many banks have this feature nowadays. 2020 saw a large increase in people using their credit cards instead of cash thanks to COVID-19 so if that was you, such features should provide a fairly accurate breakdown of your spending. You may be surprised by what you are spending your money on.

Importantly I pay off my credit card every month. I NEVER pay interest on my credit card balance. My thinking is that I am using the bank's money to temporarily pay for things but I must have the cash available or I will not use my card. I view the process as essentially an interest free short-term loan of up to 55 days. If I can't afford it now or next month, then I won't buy it. Simple.

Also investigate what awards programs there are and if they are of any value. For example, the FlyBuys program is generally considered to be unrewarding. However some programs can be great. I was part of a fantastic awards program when I was living in the UAE and I used points to pay for my return airfare from Dubai to Perth flying business class to go to my niece's wedding.

AfterPay is also a popular way for people in Australia to acquire a product immediately but pay for it later in four instalments. The repayments are interest-free but if you are late, substantial late fees apply. Just like with credit cards, this can be dangerous territory. Before signing up to such payment options, carefully look at the late fees and interest rates. At the time of writing, my bank was charging an extraordinary 20.24% interest on late payments. My latest statement indicated that if I only paid off the minimum amount owing rather than the total amount owing, it would take me 62 years and 8 months to pay off my credit card and I would pay a massive $29,915 in interest! And that is also if I don't spend any more on that credit card, ever. That is mind boggling! The lesson here is only spend what you can afford. If not, you will set yourself up for substantial financial pain.

Lazy tax

Who enjoys paying tax? I understand the importance of paying tax to fund things which have a public benefit, such as education, health and transport. But I can't say I enjoy paying tax! As Benjamin Franklin stated, in this world nothing can be said to be certain, except death and taxes. And that may be true for taxes such as income tax and transactional taxes such as stamp duty. But why are so many of us guilty of paying what's called a lazy tax? A lazy tax is the extra money we pay, mostly to an infrastructure provider, to a telecommunications provider, or to a bank simply because we're too lazy or have not bothered to shop around for a better deal. You could even call it a loyalty tax. The extra money you pay to stay loyal to the same company for years. It is the price you pay for staying with one service provider for too long, and not doing research about what's out there.

The financial year in Australia is 1 July to 30 June, and I make a point of assessing my financial situation regularly, but particularly before the end of the financial year. I have a reminder to review my financial situation at the end of April every year. This is an opportunity for me to see if I need to top up my superannuation contribution or if I should switch to another telecommunications or electricity company or health insurance provider or even adjust my level of health insurance cover. It is an annual check in to make sure that these providers are still giving me a great deal and that the service they are providing me still suits my needs. It's important to note that utilities companies and health insurance providers love to reward new customers, but existing customers don't always get access to the same deals. Shop around, haggle and bargain. Don't be afraid to ask for a better deal from your existing provider. What is the worst that can happen? They say no and if you can find a better deal elsewhere, then vote with your feet.

Ideas

Here are some ideas that may help you improve your financial situation:

1. Automate regular payments into savings, investment or superannuation accounts before you pay your bills.

2. Alter the number and scheduling of repayments on your mortgage, such as paying fortnightly instead of monthly. 26 fortnightly payments is equivalent to 13 months in repayments, so you pay an extra month off each year. For example, if your monthly repayment is currently $1,500, that equals $18,000 a year. But if you pay $750 a fortnight, that equals $19,500 a year, an extra $1,500 a year, allowing you to pay off your home faster.

3. Set a reminder on your phone or elsewhere to do an annual financial review. You should be assessing your financial situation regularly. Annually is a minimum review period, but I would recommend every three months.

4. Another trigger that you could use as a reminder to review your finances is daylight saving. If you live in an area where you have daylight saving, when you put the clocks back (usually by an hour) every autumn, use that 'extra' hour (or more) to check in on your financial status and review your accounts, debt, insurances, etc.

5. Top up your super if possible. In particular, consider pre-tax contributions such as salary sacrifice. Seek professional advice as superannuation is governed by complex rules.

6. Review and reduce or remove any subscriptions that are no longer relevant or necessary, such as streaming services, newspapers and any other form of automated payments that are not essential.

7. Seek out guidance from a financial advisor or accountant. Ask friends or other people you trust for recommendations. Do your homework on any recommendations and don't be afraid to ask lots of questions about their approach and also how they get paid.

8. Read. Research. Learn. Be a lifelong learner about all things financial.

Applying the DARE Model

Here is an example of how you can use the DARE Model to improve your financial situation:

My SMARTer lifestyle goal is…	It is 1 February 2023 and I have $2,500 extra saved in my bank account.
The SMARTer habit goal that supports my lifestyle goal is…	I will save at least $200 a month for the next 12 months.
My **Desire** for achieving this habit goal is…	10/10.
I will be **Accountable** by…	Telling my family about my goal and showing them my savings balance each month.
I will **Reward** myself for doing this habit by…	Allowing myself to binge-watch Netflix for four hours at the end of each month.
The changes I will make to my **Environment** are…	Automate a fortnightly transfer on pay day of $100 from my regular bank account to a separate savings account. Reduce my streaming services to just one subscription. Write a shopping list for groceries and stick to that list so I do not overspend. Reduce my food delivery/eating out to no more than two nights a week.

CHAPTER 10

Think

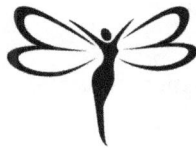

"I have no special talent. I am only passionately curious."
Albert Einstein

Introduction

In Chapter 9 – Invest, I talked about investing in yourself from a financial perspective and in Chapter 8 – Move I talked about keeping our bodies active. However, we rarely think of investing in our mental development or continuing to exercise our minds.

Have you ever forgotten where your car keys are or wondered why you walked into a particular room of your home? Have you bumped into someone at the mall who you haven't seen for a while and completely forgotten their name? I think we have all been in such situations. But what causes this? Is it decline with age? Tiredness? Or something else?

Decline in cognition

It is widely believed that normal ageing induces changes to the brain that impact some aspects of cognition, such as the speed of processing and working memory.[34] Other findings suggest that the brain reaches its peak performance between 16-25 years of age.[35] But more recent research has shown that we shouldn't accept a decline in brain function as being a normal part of ageing and that our brains are 'trainable'.

Other research has established that the more that you take care of your brain and exercise it, the more that you can slow down the brain's ageing process.[36] Brain health is also important for ensuring a better quality of life as we age.

What can affect your memory and brain function?

Some of the contributors to poor memory and decline in brain function include:

- being sleep-deprived
- being dehydrated
- chronic conditions such as high blood pressure
- smoking
- excessive alcohol consumption
- stress
- anxiety and depression
- some medications

It is interesting to note that there are a number of lifestyle factors that can contribute to cognitive decline. While brain training exercises can be helpful to help brain function, that is not the whole picture.

How can I look after my brain health?

Some of the adjustments that you can make to support your brain health have nothing to do with brain training or brain training apps. They are lifestyle changes. For example, smoking and excessive alcohol consumption have been shown as contributing factors to dementia and Alzheimer's disease. Similarly, chronic lack of sleep can contribute to cognitive decline. If you care about your mind as well as your body, consider reducing your alcohol consumption, quitting smoking and getting regular good quality sleep.

Some lifestyle factors to consider to support your brain health are:

(a) Eat a healthy diet – good nutrition is vital for optimal brain health. Diets that are high in vegetables, fruit, fish, omega-3 fatty acids (such as chia, flax and hemp seeds) and plant sources of proteins can reduce the risk of cognitive impairment and delay the onset of dementia.

(b) Be active – exercise increases the oxygenation of your blood and improves blood flow to the brain. Exercise can also help lower blood pressure and improve blood sugar and cholesterol levels. Inflammation and stress in the body are factors that adversely affect cognition. One study indicated that the more physically active adults were, the better they performed on memory tests.

(c) Be sociable – spending time with family and friends has been shown to be a contributor to good brain health. Not only does the social interaction help reduce depression (a known factor in negatively impacting cognitive ability) but it can contribute to lowering blood pressure (high blood pressure has been shown to increase the risk of cognitive decline).

(d) Get quality sleep – sleep helps to re-set the brain and allows our body and mind to heal. Sleep deprivation can hinder learning and impair cognitive performance. Getting consistent and uninterrupted sleep can assist with improved memory retention, increased alertness and higher creativity.

Brain training

While lifestyle improvements are a factor in improving your brain health, you can also train your brain. Brain exercises can improve working memory in people of all ages. The brain's plasticity – the ability of the brain to modify its own structure and essentially re-wire itself – allows it to adapt and change, even as you grow older. As you learn new things, you can create and strengthen neural pathways and networks. This helps make your brain stronger, but it can also help make it more flexible and adaptable to change.

It can also be possible to increase your intelligence to a significant degree through brain training.[37] Intelligence in this case is defined as the capacity to learn new information, retain it, then use it to solve problems or learn a new skill, rather than the ability to accumulate or memorise facts.

Mentally stimulating activities, such as reading or solving puzzles, can also play a role in delaying the onset of dementia.[38] Acquiring new knowledge also helps trigger changes in our brain that help improve our memory formation. There are numerous apps now that promote brain training, such as Elevate and Lumosity. These apps focus on skills such as memory, mathematical skills, vocabulary and focus. If you are not keen on apps, then activities such as completing jigsaw puzzles and crossword puzzles, doing Sudoku puzzles and painting and drawing can help maintain and improve cognitive function. Do not be afraid to try new things. This could be as simple as cooking a cuisine that you are not familiar with, learning to play a musical instrument or learning a second (or third or fourth) language.

> *"The beautiful thing about learning is nobody can take it away from you."*
>
> BB King

Information versus knowledge

We live in an era where we are bombarded by information on a daily basis. Sometimes it's hard to filter out the noise from matters of substance. One of the things I have focussed on in recent years is being more selective about the information that is 'pushed' to me. There is so much information that is pushed to us on social media and elsewhere that can be very distracting and that quite frankly is just noise. Ultimately, do we need to know about the infightings in the British royal family or the latest faux pas of an Instagram influencer? Sure, it can be entertaining and a silly distraction, but does it change our lives or provide us with any meaningful expansion of our knowledge? Probably not. I like to think of these types of clickbait items as junk food for the brain – something to consume in very small doses – but it should not be the majority of your diet when it comes to learning about the world around us. In my opinion, if you are serious about being the best you can be, be curious about things that really matter in our world and try not to be too distracted about the silly transient noise that is out there.

My story

I have always been a keen learner and a curious person. I am interested in the world around me and I make a point of learning something new every year. Over the past few years, this has included obtaining a Diploma in Culinary Arts and a Certificate in Governance and Risk Management. I have also learnt to surf, learnt to wakeboard, and got my motorbike licence. Apart from the personal development that these activities have afforded me, they have also enabled me to have a better understanding of the world around me and provided me with the experience to have interesting conversations with people from all backgrounds.

I also love to travel (although COVID-19 has severely curtailed this, albeit temporarily) and to meet new people and learn about other cultures. Living and working in the Middle East for ten years certainly expanded my world view and has enriched my life in so many ways. It exposed me to new perspectives and to different ways of thinking and I believe that I am a better person for it.

My personal belief is that you need to keep learning or growing, otherwise you stagnate. When an opportunity presents itself to learn and grow, I would say go for it, embrace it, and you may be surprised by where it takes you. Be curious, and the world is your oyster.

Ideas

Apart from the lifestyle factors mentioned earlier, there are things you can do that can help you expand your knowledge while strengthening your cognitive ability. Here are some ideas to inspire you:

(a) If you like watching documentaries or non-fiction, I recommend watching TED talks. TED stands for Technology,

Entertainment and Design, and the talks cover a range of informational topics from experts who are passionate about their subject matter. Topics can include things from psychology, the environment, and even space exploration. You can download the app or watch videos on YouTube.

(b) Learn to play a musical instrument. Musical training has been shown to improve brain function and long-term memory.

(c) Listen to non-fiction books and podcasts while commuting or during other 'dead' time.

(d) Do a community course or short course in an area of interest. Community colleges often have an amazing breadth of courses on offer that are inexpensive. Investigate what your local college or community centre may have on offer. They will usually have a diverse range of subjects such as photography, cake decorating, chess and business-related subjects such as social media, marketing and accounting basics.

(e) Find a brain activity you can share with others such as working on jigsaw puzzles or going to trivia nights.

(f) Try something new each year such as a new sport or a short course in an area of interest. While I am writing this book, I am looking to enrol in a course at my local community college to learn how to play the guitar.

Dare Model

Here is a sample DARE Model of what you can do to help your brain health:

My SMARTer lifestyle goal is…	It is 25 December 2022 and I am playing the guitar at AMEB (Australian Music Examinations Board) Grade 4 level.
The SMARTer habit goal that supports my lifestyle goal is…	I will practise guitar for at least 20 minutes every day.
My **Desire** for achieving this habit goal is…	8/10.
I will be **Accountable** by…	Committing to playing at least four songs in front of my family on Christmas Day 2022. Blocking out time after dinner at least five nights a week to practise guitar. Attending lessons every week and pre-paying for them.
I will **Reward** myself for doing this habit by…	Getting a manicure every two weeks when I practise at least five times a week for 20 minutes at a time.
The changes I will make to my **Environment** are…	Place the guitar in the living room so it is a visual reminder to play it instead of watching tv.

Note that this Chapter does not address head trauma or other serious conditions such as brain cancer and tumours, stroke or Parkinson's disease. Consult a medical professional if you have any concerns about your brain health.

CHAPTER 11

Restore

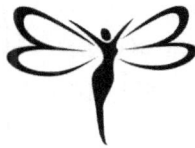

"True self care is not salt baths and chocolate cake, it is making the choice to build a life you don't need to regularly escape from."

Brianna Wiest

Introduction

What does restoration mean to you? The Macquarie Dictionary defines restore as bringing back to a state of health, soundness or vigour. We are bombarded every day with so many sounds, sights, tasks and distractions that our minds are constantly buzzing from all the sensory overload. This overstimulation can be mentally burdensome and needs to be balanced. There is a universal law of balance, which can be described by some as polarity and duality or as yin and yang. If there is an up, there is a down and if there is light, there is darkness, and one can't exist without the other. So how do we address the imbalance in our minds that our modern world places on us and restore ourselves to a state of health?

Modern life

Did you know that the average American checks their phone 52 times a day?[39] And a lot of us around the world have been guilty of doomscrolling on their devices. Doomscrolling is the practice of consuming a large volume of negative news online and continuing to scroll through bad news. There were many recent examples of this in Australia, where over the past few years we have had prolonged drought, catastrophic bushfires, extensive flooding and then COVID-19 with the loss of life and ensuing restrictions and lockdowns. It's no wonder that our mental health has taken a hit. Australian Bureau of Statistics figures indicate that the mental toll is higher in rural areas due to these cumulative stresses.[40]

Apart from the range of natural disasters we have experienced, many of us also lead hectic lives and as a result we try to do many things at once, multitasking away but not giving any one thing our full attention. It might be responding to emails while you are on a work call, it might be scrolling through social media or watching tv while eating a meal, it might be cooking dinner while trying to help your children with their homework. Switching between two or more tasks in rapid succession is a form of mental juggling and can create a mental overload. There are so many situations and examples where we try to juggle our busy adult lives by doing various tasks at the same time. Sure, that is sometimes necessary or can be effective – for example driving a car while talking to someone on a hands-free phone – but multitasking can have long-term negative impacts.

One study has shown that a person multitasking using media devices can permanently alter the structure of their brain by reductions in grey matter.[41] Other studies have shown a reduction in short-term and long-term memory as a result of multitasking.[44] Multitasking can also impact other aspects of mental health, such as heightened anxiety and chronic stress.

Research has indicated that practising mindfulness can temporarily ameliorate the negative effects on our mental health of daily stresses.[43]

"Meditation is like a gym in which you develop the powerful mental muscles of calm and insight."
Ajahn Brahm

Mindfulness, meditation and more

Meditation, gratitude lists or gratitude jars, journaling, adult colouring-in. These are some of the latest fads that are meant to provide calmness of mind. Mindfulness is also promoted as having mental health benefits and is considered to be a form of meditation as it is about being present and fully engaged in the moment. There are thousands of apps that give you the tools to practise these on your smart phone or other device. But they are not for everyone.

The first time I tried to meditate I have to admit that I found it very frustrating. I couldn't sit still and I fidgeted. I was doing a two-month meditation workshop in 2007 which was provided by my employer. A group of colleagues met weekly after work hours in one of the office conference rooms and we were taught about meditation and used the time to practise it. I remember in the first session we had to sit in a chair and close our eyes and be still and not let our minds wander. It was only for one minute but I really struggled. However, after a few months of constant practice, I found I could be calm and still for well over an hour and my mind did not wander during that time. I had made amazing progress and was proud of what I could accomplish, but overall, it wasn't a practice that I wanted to permanently introduce into my life. At the time I was of the belief that I had to meditate how monks did it, for hours in silence, to achieve calmness of mind but I subsequently discovered that for me, meditation can take many shapes. For example, I find the process of cooking to be very calming. My belief is that the process is more about calming the mind, rather than reaching a trance-like state and repeating mantras.

I have also tried journaling and gratitude lists and again, some people love these activities but they are not for me. Likewise, if you have no interest in journaling or have tried meditating but find it's not for you, then that's ok. But I would suggest trying some or all of these practices if you are new to them. I have been told by various people that they were dubious about the benefits of meditation and journaling, but when they tried it, they loved it and have kept up the practice. And if it works for you, that's great, but one size does not fit all.

But how do activities like meditation, journaling, gratitude lists and adult colouring-in provide any benefit for our mental health? Well, each of these activities are based on the principle of single-minded focus. They tend to work as calming techniques because you are focussed on that one activity only. Think of how frazzled and tired you can be when trying to juggle multiple tasks. Then think of activities where you are only focussed on one thing, such as when you are playing a sport or doing a hobby. For example, I find it impossible to think of anything else if I am doing deadlifts or doing a yoga class. I am concentrating solely on what I am doing at the time and my thoughts are in the present moment.

For me, I am of the view that mindfulness is the key to help restore the mind. Being mindful means not trying to multitask a dozen things at the same time. As a general rule, if you are looking for an activity that will help calm the mind, look for something that will focus your attention on only one thing at a time. Whether it's cooking, a bubble bath, listening to music, doing a jigsaw puzzle or swimming, find your own interpretation of 'restore'.

My story

I am a firm believer in balance and having quiet time to reflect and restore. As an introvert (according to the Myers-Briggs assessment)[44] my nature is to be reflective and I prefer to focus my energy on the inside world. I enjoy socialising, but I do find it depleting and afterwards I need time alone to restore my energy. Apart from journaling and meditation, I have also tried gratitude lists, which have been helpful, but it is not something I do every day. I have found other ways to restore and calm my mind after a hectic day. As mentioned, my favourite go-to practice is cooking a meal. Most nights, I will make a home-cooked meal, and I find the process of chopping vegetables, preparing proteins and cooking the meal as a form of meditation and flow. I get into a rhythm and focus on nothing else.

Another favourite calming experience for me is listening to music. When is the last time you listened to music and did nothing else? We tend to listen to music in the background, at a party, or in the car. But when is the last time you sat quietly and just listened to a piece of music and enjoyed it for what it is? Again, this may not be for you, but I encourage you to discover ways to help calm your mind. Remember the quote at the start of this Chapter? If chocolate cake, salt baths and candles are not for you, then find ways to create a life that provides more balance and joy.

Ideas

Let's explore some ways to help restore your mind that may work for you.

(a) Meditation – various studies have shown that meditating regularly can help to reduce stress and anxiety, improve memory, improve focus and decision-making and increase your sense of well-being. You can benefit with as little as ten minutes a day. There are some apps that can get you started, such as Calm, Headspace and Insight Timer. I suggest scheduling meditation for the same time each day. I know of a former colleague who used to sit in her car after lunch every day and meditate for ten minutes and she returned to the office feeing energised and refreshed.

(b) Journaling – this is the practice of keeping a diary or journal where you regularly write down your thoughts and feelings. By putting them to paper (or typing them in to an app), it can help give structure and meaning to your thoughts and feelings, particularly if you find that you have a lot of mental chatter. I would recommend a paper journal as the act of handwriting can force you to slow down your thoughts and the process has a calming effect. It also means you can buy an attractive journal and a fancy pen which may inspire you to write regularly, more than a smart phone would. I recommend leaving these on your bedside table and using the five minutes before turning the light off to 'dump' your thoughts for the day. This has also been shown to have sleep benefits (see Chapter 4 – Rest).

(c) Adult colouring-in – colouring books for adults have increased in popularity in recent years. They are books that contain black and white line art that you colour in with pencils, crayons or paints on paper, or digitally on e-versions. It is thought that the basic repetitive motion of colouring relaxes the brain. It also helps switch off your brain from other thoughts and requires you to be in the moment. Studies have shown that adult colouring can reduce depressive symptoms and anxiety.[45]

(d) Laughter – yes, it's true, laughter can be the best medicine! There is evidence that laughter can strengthen your immune system[46], boost your mood thanks to the release of endorphins (and the decrease in stress hormones such as cortisol and adrenaline) when you laugh, and also increase blood flow to your internal organs, as each time you laugh, you breathe more deeply, sending oxygen-rich blood through your body. It can improve the ability to see the lighter side of life in general and help manage perceptions of stress. Find a way to laugh every day, such as watching a funny show or going to a comedy gig, subscribing to a joke a day and spending time with people who put a smile on your face. You could also practise taking daily smiling selfies, even if you don't share them with anyone. You may even want to consider taking up laughter yoga (yes, it is a thing) which is a modern exercise involving prolonged voluntary laughter, as opposed to spontaneous laughter. Laughter therapy is considered as an alternative therapy for improved mental health.

(e) One of the things that can be beneficial for mental health is just to play. Remember as a child that you would spend so much time playing, but how much time do you spend as an adult engaged in playful activity? That can be something as silly as dancing a crazy dance to a favourite song, twirling a hula hoop or playing tag or hide and seek with your children.

(f) Structured 'me' time – this might be something as simple as putting time aside each day to listen to your favourite music, having a relaxing bath or reading a few pages of a book before bed.

(g) Find an enjoyable hobby or pastime that is relaxing – this could be anything from swimming to playing a musical instrument, from bushwalking to knitting. If you pursue an activity that you can share with a friend, even better, as connection is an important part of mental health (see Chapter 7 – Connect). Perhaps have a games night once a fortnight where you come together with friends and play board games or go to a trivia night with a group of friends.

"Oxygen is sustenance in a way that food can never be."
Dr Belisha Vranich

(h) Breathing exercises – most of us don't really think about our breathing but proper breathing and breath awareness have a multitude of benefits. In particular, deep breathing exercises can help reduce stress, increase energy, reduce blood pressure and improve your mental health. There are many breathing techniques to try but my favourite is a breath focus technique, where you sit comfortably in a quiet space for five minutes and breathe into the count of five, pause, and then slowly exhale to the count of five. Repeat several times.

(i) Pomodoro technique – this is a time-management technique where you break tasks down into 25-minute work intervals with a five-minute rest. The idea is that you focus on one task, and one task only, in those 25 minutes. It compels you to be mindful of the task at hand without getting distracted or trying to multitask.

(j) Do nothing – yes that's right, sometimes it is good for the brain to fully shut down. Also take the pressure off yourself when you go about your day. Go for a walk but don't count your steps. Cook a meal but don't feel pressured to produce a masterpiece. Give yourself some slack and remove the mental pressure you put on yourself.

(k) Opt-in to news services for only a set period each day and be intentional in how you access news. Seek out quality news sources that focus on thoughtful consumption, rather than 'clickbait' articles that encourage an emotional response.

(l) Counselling – sometimes a life event or chronic mental distress may require professional support. When I separated from my now ex-husband, I was an emotional mess. What helped me get through the emotional upheaval at the time was talking to a counsellor. One of the benefits of seeing a professional was she didn't know my ex-husband so she was neutral (unlike friends and family) and she was skilled at asking me the right questions. Being able to open up to her lifted a lot of mental burden and negative emotion. If you are in distress, then seek professional help. Organisations in Australia such a Beyond Blue and Lifeline can offer support if you are experiencing a personal crisis.

Applying the DARE Model

Here is how you might apply the DARE Model to create habits to help you restore:

My SMARTer lifestyle goal is…	It is 1 March 2022 and I am practising hatha yoga for at least four hours a week.
The SMARTer habit goal that supports my lifestyle goal is…	I will attend yoga classes at my gym every Tuesday, Thursday and Sunday.
My **Desire** for achieving this habit goal is…	8/10.
I will be **Accountable** by…	Committing to a gym membership. Booking into classes online a week ahead of time.
I will **Reward** myself for doing this habit by…	Buying a new yoga mat when I attend yoga classes at least three times a week for the first month and buying new leggings when I attend yoga classes three times a week after the first two months.
The changes I will make to my **Environment** are…	Place my yoga clothes, mat and gym bag out in the evenings before yoga class.

CHAPTER 12

Go!

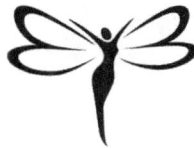

"Opportunities are like sunrises. If you wait too long, you miss them."

William Arthur Ward

Many of us bumble through life on autopilot. We go to work, we come home, we look after family, we binge-watch Netflix on weekends and eat junk food and drink excessive amounts of alcohol, and then we repeat, week in week out, month after month, year after year. We fall into bad habits like lack of sleep, poor diet and lack of exercise. We are tired but know we can do better and feel better but don't know how to make the shift to a more positive and rewarding life.

Imagine your ideal life. What would it look like? How would it make you feel? What is stopping you from making positive changes in your life?

Hopefully, this book has inspired you in some ways to make some positive changes in your life and has helped you establish positive habits that stick.

So what are you waiting for? Go!

About the Author

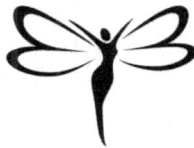

"I help professional women create positive lifestyle habits that stick."

Dee Matlok was born and raised in the Illawarra region of New South Wales, Australia and graduated from the University of Wollongong with a Bachelor of Laws and Bachelor of Commerce. She has more than 25 years' experience as a successful international lawyer and knowledge manager, having worked and lived in the Middle East for 10 years. She has expertise in commercial contracts, contract negotiations, integrity and risk management. In 2016, her legal team won the Asia-MENA In-House Community Team of the Year award for the Energy & Natural Resources sector and were finalists in the Infrastructure, Utilities and Energy Team of the Year at the Australian Corporate Counsel Awards in 2018. She was a committee member of the Australian Business Council in Dubai and led the review of that organisation's constitution in 2013. Dee also has a Certificate in Governance and Risk Management and was a Fellow of the Governance Institute of Australia. She has experience in the fields of knowledge management and technology, and she is always striving to find better and more efficient ways for individuals and organisations to do business.

The pressures of professional life led Dee to increase her knowledge and awareness about the importance of being committed to regular exercise, maintaining a healthy and balanced diet, and practising mindfulness, to support and enable excellence in her professional and personal life. With a lifelong love of learning, Dee has a Certificate in Nutrition, a Diploma in Food Preparation and Cooking (Culinary Arts) (Distinction) and a Certificate in Exercise Science (Personal Trainer) and is studying to become an accredited Life Coach, with completion scheduled for 2021.

Dee is an avid runner and triathlete, and she has completed several long-distance triathlons and multi-day running events in some of the toughest terrains in the world, including the Sahara and Gobi Deserts. As part of that experience, she has appeared in various media, including newspapers and magazines in the Middle East, as well as participating in various television and radio interviews. She was a guest speaker at the "Inspire Talks" sessions, a series of talks across the United Arab Emirates to inspire high school and university age women to strive to achieve academic, professional and personal excellence. She is committed to raising awareness about mental health and wellness issues, which led to her nomination for the Australian of the Year Award in 2014.

In her spare time, Dee enjoys cooking, lifting weights, travelling and being a servant to her fur baby cat, Phoenix.

Website	www.deematlok.com
Facebook	Dee Matlok author
LinkedIn	Dee (Doris) Matlok
Instagram	Dee_Matlok
TikTok	Dee_Matlok

AS READ IN AND HEARD ON:

ABB news
Abu Dhabi Classic FM
Ahlan Live
Arabian Gazette
City 7 TV
Dubai Eye Radio
Dubai PR Network
Emirates News
Esquire ME
Gulf News
InnerFight podcast with Marcus Smith
Inspire Talks with Hermoine Macura
Outdoor UAE
Seven Days newspaper
Shape ME magazine
Switch your Sitch podcast with Katie Turner
The National newspaper
The Sweat Shop
Times of Oman
Viva Middle East

Acknowledgements

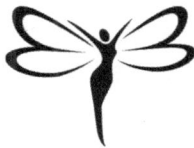

I was fortunate to have grown up in a family with a mum who is a very strong, self-sufficient and independent woman and I have inherited many of those traits from her. She is an amazing cook, which I am sure is largely due to her Austrian heritage and meant that we always had healthy home-cooked meals in our home when I was growing up. She is also super sensible with money. So, I had a good start in life because she taught me some important life skills and habits. Thank you. I love you very much. My stepdad has also been an amazing figure in my life. Always kind, curious and happy to know what is going on in my life. Thank you for your support. I love you too.

A big shout out to Natasa Denman and her extraordinary team. This book would not have been possible without them.

Lots of hugs and love to my amazing support crew – Kate, Maegan, Luke, Liz U, Mark, Ileana, Jaymi, Michelle, Hermoine, and Geoff. You guys are amazing and I wouldn't have got this far without you.

Bonus Offers

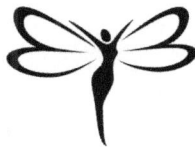

To get your downloadable, modifiable DARE Model template, go to www.deematlok.com

You can also access an array of other resources from the website, such as recipes for weeknight meals that are quick, tasty and healthy.

Are you looking for a speaker for your next event? Dee is an engaging and inspiring speaker who shares her knowledge and experience in a warm, practical and accessible way.

Dee is also available for one on one and group coaching.

Appendix

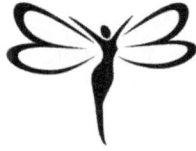

My SMARTer lifestyle goal is…	
The SMARTer habit goal that supports my lifestyle goal is…	
My **Desire** for achieving this habit goal is…	
I will be **Accountable** by…	
I will **Reward** myself for doing this habit by…	
The changes I will make to my **Environment** are…	

Endnotes

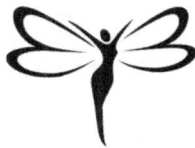

1 Duhigg, Charles. The Power of Habit: Why We Do What We Do in Life and Business. New York: Random House, 2012.

2 Clear, James. Atomic habits: tiny changes, remarkable results : an easy & proven way to build good habits & break bad ones. New York : Avery, an imprint of Penguin Random House, 2018.

3 Dr Rangan Chattergee, mailing list

4 The original concept of a wheel of life is attributed to Paul J Meyer who was a coaching industry pioneer.

5 What Is Happiness and Why Is It Important? Cortney E Ackerman MA, Positivepsychology.com, 31 October 2020

6 B Sahakian and JN LaBuzetta, Bad Moves: How decision making goes wrong, and the ethics of smart drugs, OUP Oxford, 2013.

7 Wansink, Brian and Jeffery Sobal (2007), "Mindless Eating: The 200 Daily Food Decisions We Overlook," Environment and Behavior, 39:1 (January), 106-23

8 Effects of insufficient sleep on circadian rhythmicity and expression amplitude of the human blood transcriptome, Carla S. Möller-Levet, Simon N. Archer, Giselda Bucca, Emma E. Laing, Ana Slak, Renata Kabiljo, June C. Y. Lo, Nayantara Santhi, Malcolm von Schantz, Colin P. Smith, and Derk-Jan Dijk, Proceedings of the National Academy of Sciences of the United States of America, 19 March 2013.

9   One night of sleep loss impairs innovative thinking and flexible decision making, Y Harrison 1, J A Horne, Organizational Behavior and Human Decision Processes. 1999 May;78(2):128-45

10 Brief communication: Sleep curtailment in healthy young men is associated with decreased leptin levels, elevated ghrelin levels, and increased hunger and appetite, Karine Spiegel 1, Esra Tasali, Plamen Penev, Eve Van Cauter, Annals of Internal Medicine, 2004 Dec 7;141(11):846-50.

11 Husby R, Lingjaerde O. Prevalence of reported sleeplessness in northern Norway in relation to sex, age and season. Acta Psychiatr. Scand. 1990;81:542–547; Arendt, Josephine. Biological Rhythms During Residence in Polar Regions. Chronobiol Int. 2012 May; 29(4): 379–394

12 The Biology of REM Sleep, John Peever and Patrick M. Fuller, Current Biology, 11 January 2016 26(1): R34–R35.

13 Chamara Visanka Senaratna, Dallas R. English, Dianne Currier, Jennifer L. Perret, Adrian Lowe, Caroline Lodge, Melissa Russell, Sashane Sahabandu, Melanie C. Matheson, Garun S. Hamilton, Shyamali C. Dharmage. Sleep apnoea in Australian men: disease burden, co-morbidities, and correlates from the Australian longitudinal study on male health. BMC Public Health. 2016; 16(Suppl 3): 51–61. Published online 2016 Oct 31.

14 ABS 2018. National Health Survey: First Results, 2017–18. ABS cat. no. 4364.0.55.001. Canberra: Australian Bureau of Statistics.

15 Marie-Pierre St-Onge, Anja Mikic, Cara E Pietrolungo, Effects of Diet on Sleep Quality, Advances in Nutrition, Volume 7, Issue 5, September 2016, Pages 938–949, https://doi.org/10.3945/an.116.012336

16 National Health and Medical Research Council of Australia. Clinical Practice Guidelines for the Management of Overweight and Obesity in Adults, Adolescents and Children in Australia. Australian Government, 2013.

17 Peirce, JM, Alviña, K. The role of inflammation and the gut microbiome in depression and anxiety. J Neuro Res. 2019; 97: 1223– 1241. https://doi.org/10.1002/jnr.24476

18 Ruth Ann Carpenter, Carrie E Finley. Health Eating Every Day, 2nd edition. HumanKinetics, 2017.

19 Finder analysis of Australian Bureau of Statistics 2021, www.finder.com.au

20 Australian Bureau of Statistics Household Expenditure Survey 2015-2016.

21 Australian Institute of Health and Welfare 2021. Alcohol, tobacco & other drugs in Australia. Cat. no. PHE 221. Canberra: AIHW. Viewed 17 April 2021, https://www.aihw.gov.au/reports/alcohol/alcohol-tobacco-other-drugs-australia

22 https://www.breastcancer.org/risk/factors/alcohol#:~:text=Alcohol%20can%20increase%20levels%20of,higher%20risk%20of%20breast%20cancer.

23 Holt-Lunstad J, Smith TB, Layton JB (2010) Social Relationships and Mortality Risk: A Meta-analytic Review. PLoS Med 7(7): e1000316. https://doi.org/10.1371/journal.pmed; Betty Pfefferbaum, M.D., J.D., and Carol S. North, M.D., M.P.E. Mental Health and the Covid-19 Pandemic. N Engl J Med 2020; 383:510-512 DOI: 10.1056/NEJMp2008017; Jean M. Twenge (2013) Does Online Social Media Lead to Social Connection or Social Disconnection? Journal of College and Character, 14:1, 11-20, DOI:10.1515/jcc-2013-0003

24 https://pineapplegeorge.com/2019/01/22/it-has-to-start-with-you-the-incredible-story-of-kotti/

25 A great book on this topic is How to Think About Exercise by Damon Young.

26 NAB Australian Wellbeing Survey for Q4 2019

27 How to prove the gender pay gap to a non-believer, Jamila Rizvi, The Sydney Morning Herald, March 5, 2019

28 How much money should you have in your superannuation by age, Kathy Skantzos, news.com.au, 4 January 2021

29 Australian census, 2016.

30 Robert Kiyosaki. Rich Dad, Poor Dad: What the Rich Teach Their Kids About Money That the Poor and Middle Class Do Not! Plata Publishing, 2017.

31 Robert Kiyosaki. Rich Dad, Poor Dad: What the Rich Teach Their Kids About Money That the Poor and Middle Class Do Not! Plata Publishing, 2017.

32 Scott Pape. The Barefoot Investor; The Only Money Guide You'll Ever Need. Wiley, 2020.

33 Daryl Guppy, Trend Trading: A Seven-step Approach to Success. Wiley, 2004

34 Reuter-Lorenz PA, Lustig C. Brain aging: reorganizing discoveries about the aging mind. Curr Opin Neurobiol. 2005;15(2):245–251. [PubMed]

35 Baltes, P. et al. (1999), Lifespan Psychology: Theory and Application to Intellectual Functioning. Annual Review of Psychology 50: 471-507

36 Murman DL. (2015). The Impact of Age on Cognition. Seminars in hearing, 36(3), 111–121. https://doi.org/10.1055/s-0035-1555115

37 Susanne M. Jaeggi, M. B. (2008). Improving Fluid intelligence With Training on Working Memory. Proceedings of the National Academy of Sciences. doi: 10.1073/pnas.0801268105

38 https://www.mayoclinic.org/diseases-conditions/dementia/symptoms-causes/syc-20352013

39 Deloitte's 2018 Global Mobile Consumer Survey.

40 https://mindframemedia.imgix.net/assets/src/uploads/ABS-Causes-of-Death-data-2019_Australian-state-and-territories-summary.pdf

41 Higher Media Multi-Tasking Activity Is Associated with Smaller Gray-Matter Density in the Anterior Cingulate Cortex. Kep Kee Loh, Ryota Kanai PLoS One. 2014; 9(9): e106698. Published online 2014 Sep 24.

42 Media multitasking and memory: Differences in working memory and long-term memory. Melina R Uncapher, Monica K Thieu, Anthony D Wagner. Psychon Bull Rev 2016 Apr 23, 489-490.

43 Gorman, T., Green, C. Short-term mindfulness intervention reduces the negative attentional effects associated with heavy media multitasking. Sci Rep 6, 24542 (2016). https://doi.org/10.1038/srep24542

44 https://www.myersbriggs.org/my-mbti-personality-type/mbti-basics/

45 Jayde A. M Flett, Celia Lie, Benjamin C Riordan, Laura M Thompson, Tamlin S Conner & Harlene Hayne (2017) Sharpen Your Pencils: Preliminary Evidence that Adult Coloring Reduces Depressive Symptoms and Anxiety, Creativity Research Journal, 29:4, 409-416, DOI: 10.1080/10400419.2017.1376505

46 Yim J. Therapeutic benefits of laughter in mental health: a theoretical review. The Tohoku Journal of Experimental Medicine. 2016;239(3):243–249. doi: 10.1620/tjem.239.243. - DOI - PubMed

Notes

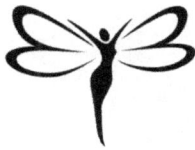

_____

_____

_____

_____

_____

_____

_____

_____